How To Train And Care For Your Cockapoo Puppy

Complete dog training guide for beginners including House & Potty Training, Crate and Recall Training, Separation Anxiety, Health and Breed Information

Helen Sutherland

To Poppy, Holly and Rowan

Thanks for all your lessons

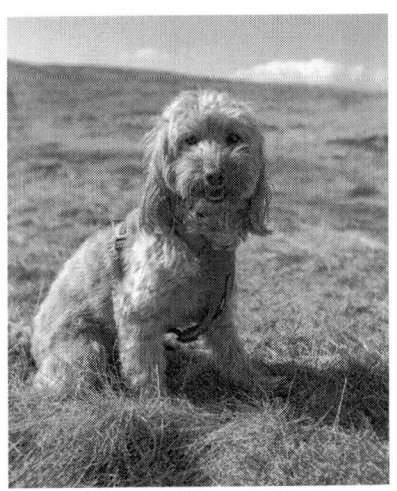

Poppy

Contents

Introduction   ix

1. A BRIEF HISTORY OF COCKAPOOS   1
   Related Breeds   1
   The Poodle   3
   The Cocker Spaniel   5
   Cockapoos   6
   What does F1 and F2 mean?   8

2. HEALTH, CARE AND WELLBEING   13
   Hybrid Vigor   13
   Ears and Skin   14
   Eyes   16
   Teeth   17
   Nails   17
   Coat And Grooming   17
   Dew claws   18
   Loss of Blood/Weight   20
   Von Willebrand Disease   20
   Elbow and Hip Dysplasia   21
   Eating poop   21
   To Spay or to Neuter your dog ?   22

3. PLANNING AHEAD   26

4. WELCOME HOME   30
   Socialization   31
   Vaccinations over the first year   33

5. HOUSE AND POTTY TRAINING   35
   How long can a puppy wait for the toilet   36
   Puppy Pads   37
   How to manage their potty training   38

Your schedule   43
Sleep   45

6. CRATE TRAINING   49
Introducing your puppy to the crate   50
Size and Types of Crate   54

7. FOOD AND FEEDING   56
What to feed them   56
How much to feed   59
What not to feed - dangerous foods for
your dog   60

8. CHEWING AND MOUTHING   63
Mouthing   63
Chewing   66

9. TRAINING AT HOME   70
Basic Training   73
The fundamental cues   76
Summary and the 10 steps for basic recall   81
Leash training   81

10. RECALL TRAINING   83
Cues   83
Training Outside   87
Using the long-line   89
Using a Clicker   92
Distractions   95
Proofing   96
Emergency stop   97
What not to do   99

11. PARK LIFE   101
Other dogs and their communication signals   103
How dogs greet each other   104
How to interact with humans   107
Games   107

12. GENERAL TRAINING TIPS   110
  Introducing her to the sitter   110
  Introducing her to a new home with dogs   110
  Activities to avoid until adulthood   111
  Excessive Barking   111

13. SEPARATION ANXIETY   114
  Dogs are not the same   116
  Signs Of Separation Anxiety   117
  Signs of anxiety   120
  Punishment Won't Work   121
  Preparation   123
  Getting her used to not being beside you   123
  Leaving and returning   126
  Leaving when using a crate   129
  10 Steps to help Separation Anxiety   131

14. HOW TO FIND A BREEDER   132
  How to recognise a puppy farm   133

15. CONCLUSION AND SUMMARY   136
16. NEED MORE HELP?   138

  Leave A Review   141
  More Books From Twenty Dogs   143
  Resources and Citations   145

Introduction

Who doesn't love a Cockapoo?! Whether you are already a dog owner that has another type of dog or whether you aren't a dog owner - it is impossible not to love this cheeky, beautiful bundle of fur.

Unlike some other breeds they don't shed too much, they are generally healthy, with a long lifespan, and they are a great choice of dog for both single parent owners or as a family puppy.

But don't be fooled by that gorgeous little innocent face. As my grandmother would say, this little bundle of joy is a 'little tear-away'. That personality is big! Loving, stubborn, playful, possessive, loyal, joyful (some would say an enthusiastic joker), and strong-willed but she is also prone to separation anxiety. And in a big way, but this might depend on the number of people in your household. And these bundles of joy are intelligent with a mind that seems to work at a hundred miles an hour.

Introduction

When you are writing about dogs, the modus operandi is to use the term 'He', but in this book it just has to be 'She'. The ones that are in my life are mostly all girls but if you have, or are thinking about, a boy, the training and advice is the same.

I know four of these dogs extremely well. Poppy, Holly, Rowan and Macey (Macey is actually a Schitzpoo but many of the characteristics are similar). Poppy and Holly are the perfect specimens of the Cockapoo. They display both the very best and the most annoying traits and both are remarkably similar. Poppy has helped me with this book in almost every conceivable way and has allowed me to include all of the most typical training needs and problems that you will have.

I have done lots of dog training over the years and my own dogs (particularly one of them) lead me to taking accreditations in dog training. The one I am most passionate about is recall and recall training is really important for these dogs.

Separation anxiety is also something I have had to deal with and so has Poppy's mum. There isn't too much practical training you can do for separation in terms of classes, but there are some really simple things that you need to do every day to ease this problem. And it is a problem - for both you and your puppy. Cockapoos need separation training from the very start.

Cockapoos are happy and outgoing, which makes them sociable with people and other dogs and they make excellent family companions - they have been bred to be companion dogs. They are affectionate and loyal and love to be cuddled and love attention. On top of this they are smart and easily trainable but they can bark a lot.

However, it is because of their need for attention and companionship that they can be clingy and experience separation anxiety easily which is why, if you spend any significant time outside of the home, you need to train them how to be left alone.

They also get bored easily if they don't get enough attention - they have smart and active minds. When this happens they can become destructive and may bark at you. Therefore, it is important to keep her exercised and give her some mental stimulation every day. These bundles of love and joy need you to spend time with them.

Finally, the Cockapoo is sometimes said to be hypoallergenic. All dogs produce dander which is simply dead skin cells. It is these that can cause allergic reactions. There is no scientific evidence that any breed or cross breed is more or less allergenic than any other dog. Some people with allergies may react less severely to particular dogs, but no-one can guarantee that a dog is hypoallergenic. What will help, is that they shed less than many other dog types such as German Shepherd Dogs or Cocker Spaniels.

This book will start with the breed itself. Where she comes from and the traits of the breeds from which she came. One of those breeds is the Cocker Spaniel. I have two Cockers and it's hard not to notice where the similarities are.

I will also cover how to find a reputable dealer along with the common health problems.

In summary, our little Cockapoos have big personalities, they are highly intelligent, loving, loyal, easy-to-train, agile, and low-shedding dogs. They are usually quite healthy, and with an estimated life expectancy of between 13-15 years but don't be surprised if your pup gets to the ripe old age of 20. It certainly won't be boring!

Chapter 1
A brief history of Cockapoos

B efore we begin it is useful to take a brief look at most of the well known poodle crosses. This book is about Cockapoos but if you are thinking about a Cockapoo then you will no doubt have heard about Cavapoos and Shih-Poos. We have a Shih Poo in our family, called Macey and I know both a Cavapoos and a few Cockapoos very well. In truth, for the uninitiated, it is hard to tell them all apart but there are some subtle differences.

Related Breeds

Very briefly the following pages will provide an overview of these related breeds and then we take a look at our Cockapoo herself.

The Cavapoo is a cross between the Poodle and the Cavalier King Charles Spaniel and they became popular in the late 1990's. While most of the world calls this breed a Cavapoo, in Australia it is known as a Cavoodle. They look a lot like the

Cockapoo only smaller (depending on your choice of Cockapoo).

Both of these dogs have coats that are prone to matting and grooming is needed every few weeks. Most owners will do this general grooming at home. Try to focus on the eyes, paws, and around the tail. Both will need a thorough groom and shampoo every 5-7 weeks. Because the Cavapoo has a thinner coat the knotting in Cavapoos is slightly worse than the Cockapoo but easy to prevent by brushing every few days.

Cavapoos are mostly small dogs that stand around 9 to 14 inches at the shoulder and you can expect a weight range from 8-25 pounds. Cockapoos are produced in four various size categories, depending on the size of the poodle parent (there is more detail on this later).

A Cockapoo has longer ears compared to the Cavapoo. This trait occurs is a result of genes inherited from the Cocker Spaniel.

Now to their noses! The Cockapoo has a more elongated nose than the Cavapoo. The Cavapoo inherits the skull shape and nose of the Cavalier King Charles Spaniel and the Cockapoo inherits her shape from the Cocker Spaniel which means the main difference in appearance between Cavapoo and Cockapoo is the skull shape beneath the hair.

If you are wondering about this, then you might be interested to know that dog skull shapes are split into 3 types. The Cocker Spaniel's skull is known as 'mesocephalic'. It is the most proportional of the three skull shapes and is also known as 'square-skulled'. There is a good reason for this shape. It is the broader snouts and larger nasal cavities that give them their scenting capabilities.

The King Charles Spaniel skull shape falls into the brachy-cephalic type. This is often thought to be the cutest shape for dog owners. It is a relatively broad and short skull type with the breadth at least 80% of the length of the muzzle. History suggests that these dogs were known as 'fighting dogs' and that the reason for the shape was to achieve stronger jaws.

The Shih Poo is possibly less well known and is a cross between the Shih Tzu and Toy Poodle. Shih-Poos also go by the names Shoodle or Pooshi but should not be confused with the Poo-Shi, the Poodle/Shiba Inu mix.

They tend to be 8 to 18 inches in height and weigh 8 to 18 pounds. Perhaps the main thing to note about Shih Poos is that they are particularly good for seniors as well as a family. Shih Poos are ideally better if you have some experience of dogs, although they are not generally high energy pups they can be harder to train. They are very affectionate but don't tolerate other dogs too well and, like their Cavapoo and Cockerpoo cousins, they are playful and can be prone to separation anxiety.

The Poodle

Your Cockapoo comes from the parental line that includes the Poodle (either first generation or longer). It is useful to know a little bit about Poodles. These are fascinating dogs and really deserve much more space but I have included just a few high-lights that will be interesting for Cockapoo owners.

The Poodle is a breed of water dog and it is divided into four varieties based on size, the Standard Poodle, Medium Poodle, Miniature Poodle and Toy Poodle. The Medium Poodle is not always recognised as a breed type.

Poodles are known for being one of the most intelligent of all dog breeds, their athleticism and their sociable nature and they make great companion dogs (like the Cockapoo) and this is one of the reasons that they became Circus dogs in France. It might also be one of the reason that your Cockapoo likes to do tricks!

Both Germany and France are often cited as where the Poodle originates and in Germany they were known as Pudels and in France, they were called a Caniche. It is believed that the Miniature Poodle comes from the French Circus Poodles because it was easier to transport smaller dogs and, in 1907, the Miniature Poodles became even smaller with the introduction of the Toy Poodle. This was because the smaller dogs were believed to make better companion dogs.

The largest Poodle, the Standard Poodle, was used by fowl hunters to retrieve game from water (similar to Cocker Spaniels who were originally used for 'flushing out' birds). In fact, the name Pudel translates into the old German word that means "to splash". This means that when you hear that the Poodle is a hunting dog it is most likely referring to the Standard Poodle. It also explains why your Cockapoo will love the water and love to swim (but don't confuse loving water with loving a bath - Holly hates her bath!).

In terms of their famous coast, it is commonly believed that the Poodle does not shed but in fact they do. Rather than the fur coming off the dog it gets tangled up in the surrounding hair and this is what leads to matting without proper care. This will be a familiar experience for Cockapoo owners. Her hair will matt easily and you need to pay attention to her grooming.

The Cocker Spaniel

I have two Cocker Spaniels - both Working Cockers.

The history of Cocker Spaniels dates back to at least the fourteenth century but they were not recognised as a breed until the 1800's.

There are two main types (if you exclude the Working Cocker) - the English and the American Cocker and both types are used to breed with Poodles to create our Cockapoos.

As you would expect they both share similar heritage but the English Cocker came first. Originally known as the Cocking Spaniel, the English Cocker Spaniel was grouped with a number of other spaniel hunting breeds which were separated by type and hunting ability.

The Cocking Spaniel, the real ancestor for our Cockapoo line, was known for his smaller size and the way he hunted birds.

It was not until the 20th Century that American enthusiasts of the English Cocker Spaniel decided to breed a companion dog of comparable temperament and beauty. This smaller dog was bred to be more relaxed and to have a more family-oriented personality.

The American Cocker reminds me of the German Shepherd Dog where their mission in life is to please his family and to be with them as much as possible. It is this trait that can lead to separation anxiety and this trait is also seen in Cockapoos (and GSD's). The English Cocker, while undoubtedly a family-loving dog, tends to be more energetic with more of a prey drive.

Across both Poodles and Spaniels the most common problem is one of ear infections and this is a problem that our Cockapoos can also experience - mainly due to their longer ears.

There is also some evidence that liver disease is becoming more common in Cocker Spaniels. They take two forms: chronic active hepatitis and copper toxicosis. It is not yet known if these conditions are genetic. It would be good practice to ask your Cockapoo breeder about the parent Cocker's liver history.

Cockapoos

Cockapoos, also known as Cockerpoos, Cockerdoodles or Spoodles in Australia, and are cross-breed from Cocker Spaniels and Poodles.

The Cockapoo was once described as a designer dog but that term is rarely used these days. Designer dogs were, and are, hybrids but the Cockapoo is an 'old' hybrid. We don't really know how they started, whether it was an accident or a love affair between a Poodle and a Cocker who's eyes met across a crowded dog park (or bowl), but it worked, and they have been popular since the late 1950's and 1960s. They are the result of crossbreeding rather than inbreeding which means their genetics are often enhanced - this is known as hybrid vigor.

Inbreeding tends to amplify weaker traits, while crossbreeding can help avoid certain undesirable traits because the crossbreeding adds strength to the gene pool. In other words, recessive genes may not be expressed as often when mixing breeds.

The AKC does not recognize Cockapoos as a breed group but some dog clubs are carefully breeding consecutive generations to eventually establish cockapoos as a recognized breed. The efforts to establish the breed standard will need agreement on what the 'true breed' of a Cockapoo should be because a 'true breed' is one that produces offspring with consistent traits.

I have no idea how this will work out and if it really matters. But, in terms of 'breeding' and being 'true bred' I can see a few hurdles. Not least that no-one can agree on what this should be.

Some want to make the Cockapoo a purebred dog and use multigeneration crossing, while other breeders prefer the basic Poodle/Cocker cross.

The Cockapoo Club of America formed in 1999 promotes breeding multigenerational Cockapoos to each other as opposed to creating new first generations, because this technique is supposed to help puppies maintain the desired qualities that aren't seen in all first-generation dogs.

The American Cockapoo Club don't mix generations and don't breed a Cockapoo back to a Poodle or a Cocker Spaniel. They too have a breed standard, and their goal is "to see genuine Cockapoos bred with lines that can be traced back to their originating roots of AKC/CKC Cocker Spaniels and AKC/CKC Poodles."

The North American Cockapoo Registry provides certification for Cockapoos who are the results of first- through sixth-generation breedings. The Registry stipulates that "a true Cockapoo is ONLY a purposeful, planned crossing of a purebred Cocker Spaniel with a purebred Poodle."

If you are confused, so is everyone else.

First generational is a puppy that comes from a Cocker and a Poodle. Multi generational is complicated and can be a Cockapoo with a Spaniel or Poodle and then their offspring - or a cockapoo with a cockapoo.

It is complicated to explain in words and the diagram below might help to give you a general idea. More practically, it matters more if you want to breed your Cockapoo. In this case, you will need to know what 'generation' you are breeding.

What does F1 and F2 mean?

The Terms F_1 and F_2 and so on are used to describe what generational cross a Cockapoo is.

A first generation Cockapoo, or F_1, is the offspring of a Poodle and Spaniel.i.e. They are 50% Poodle and 50% Spaniel.

A second generation Cockapoo, or F_2, is the result of a first generation Cockapoo breeding with another first generation Cockapoo.

If a Cockapoo is bred with a Cocker Spaniel or a Poodle then the offspring are given a 'b' suffix which tells us that the offspring have been bred back to the original breed. The table that follows provides and example of Cockapoo generations.

Cocker Spaniel	and	Poodle	F1
F1 Cockapoo	and	F1 Cockapoo	F2
F2 Cockapoo	and	F2 Cockapoo	F3
F3 Cockapoo	and	F3 Cockapoo	F4
F1 Cockapoo	and	Cocker Spaniel or Poodle	F1b
F2 Cockapoo	and	Cocker Spaniel or Poodle	F2b
F1b Cockapoo	and	F1 Cockapoo	F2b
F1b Cockapoo	and	F2 Cockapoo	F2b
F1b Cockapoo	and	F3 Cockapoo	F2b

Example of Cockapoo Generations

The important point to note here is that you really don't know what a Cockapoo will look like until she is around 6 weeks old. An F1 or an F2 can, and do, look the same. Even within an F1 and an F2 generation you are going to get a mix of different coats, some will be straighter and some more wooly and curly.

Your Cockapoo will either be a mix of Poodle (the type will depend on the size of the mother, assuming the Poddle is the father) and an English or American Cocker Spaniel, although the American Cocker tends to be the most common.

The miniature poodle is normally paired with an English Cocker and a toy poodle is often used with an American cocker spaniel. This can vary but the important thing is that the sizes are matched to ensure the mother does not have difficulty in giving birth due to over large puppies. The Poodle is often the father but this isn't a golden rule as the Poodle can be the mother too.

The main difference between American Cocker and the English Cocker is that the English Cocker has a strong prey drive and may be more inclined to follow a scent meaning that she could be more tempted to wander off to follow that scent.

As we already know, Cocker Spaniels have a past as working dogs which means that your Cockapoo will love a game of fetch due to this working dog heritage. Like their DNA heritage, Cockapoos are highly intelligent and eager to please – a combination that makes them easy to train. They thrive on attention (the toy poodle heritage) and will love the time spent with you during training sessions. If your Cockapoo is the result of a Working Cocker cross she will have more energy and be more agile than a Cockappoo who's parent is a Show Cocker - these pups tend to be calmer, but you can never be 100% sure.

In terms of their coat color, Cockapoos coats will vary in color in the same way that Spaniels and Poodles do and it will depend on the parents from which they were bred. The color will typically range from black, cream, brown, tan, white and sometimes a combination of these colors.

The texture will vary anywhere between, and including, silky smooth to tight curls.

As you would expect, Cockapoos come in different sizes which are remarkably similar to the Poodle size types, and the parents' genetics determine what size (and color) it will be.

Generally speaking, they come in four different size categories as follows:-

The Teacup Toy - weighs less than 6 pounds and stands less than 10 inches in high.

The Toy Cockapoo - the larger ones can weigh up to 12 pounds and reach 11 inches tall.

The Miniature Cockapoo - weighs 13 to 25 pounds and ranges between 11 and 15 inches tall. This is the most commonly seen Cockapoo.

The Standard or Maxi Cockapoo - weighs more than 25 pounds and should be at least 16 inches in height.

The following table indicates height and weight range

	Standard/ Maxi	Miniature	Toy	Teacup
Height	16 – 22 inches	11 – 15 inches	10 – 11 inches	Under 10 inches
Weight	Over 25 lbs	13 – 25 lbs	6 – 12 lbs	Under 6 lbs
Age when full grown	12 – 14 months	9 – 12 months	7 – 9 months	5 – 7 months

Cockapoo Height and Weight Range

Poodles have a reputation for being hypoallergenic, meaning that they can be tolerated by people who have allergies to dogs and because Cockapoos have the Poodle in their heritage, they are sometimes promoted as being hypoallergenic. But allergies are not caused by a particular dog coat type but by dander which is simply the dead skin cells that are shed by all dogs and people.

There is no scientific evidence that any breed or cross breed is more or less allergenic than any other dog. Some people with allergies may react less severely to particular dogs, but no-one can guarantee that a dog is hypoallergenic. It is true to say that they are low shedding and that the might be low shedders of dander but it is not true to say that they shed no dander.

Cockapoos do need their coat to be looked after but not at the level of grooming that is required by a Poodle. They will need frequent grooming and, ideally, regular visits to a dog groomer.

Cockapoos are generally known to have moderate energy levels but they do need daily exercise. I know a few owners who would disagree with the 'moderate' energy description! Just ensure that you can give them a good walk each day and play games with them or teach them tricks - remember, they are highly intelligent dogs and they like to use their brains.

Chapter 2
Health, Care and Wellbeing

I n this chapter we cover the main areas of your Cockapoos general care as well as highlighting some of the most common health problem that your Cockapoo might experience at some point in her life. Don't worry too much because, overall, Cockapoos are healthy and don't have many, or any, inherent health issues.

Hybrid Vigor

Hybrid Vigor will be a term that you hear when you are talking to breeders about Cockapoos. Hybrid Vigor is to do with DNA. The genes that DNA contains include alleles and these alleles can contain disorders and diseases.

Essentially, an allele will not express itself if there is only one copy of that allele in a gene. It means that it won't be 'active' and affect the health of your dog if there is only one copy rather than two. One allele comes from the mother and one allele comes from the father.

Purebred dogs come from a narrow gene pool of DNA - and certainly a narrower gene pool than that of a hybrid dog like your Cockapoo. Hybrids, in effect, provide the opportunity to widen the gene pool that provides more 'good' allele options from which to select. This means that the breeder can select a Cocker Spaniel and Poodle and 'iron-out' any historic disorders or diseases from each breed line. The Animal Health Trust explained this in a press release, "Because of the small gene pool in purebred dogs, inherited diseases resulting from single gene mutations are more likely to occur than in their cross bred cousins". It means that, if both parents suffer from the same condition, the pups could be affected.

There's good evidence, for example, that Labradoodles are just as likely to suffer hip dysplasia as their purebred parent breeds. The breed mean hip score for Labradors is 15 and for Standard Poodles it is 14 while the Labradoodle's average hip score is 14".

It all means that hybrid dogs, on average, should be healthier than the purebred breed from which they came, but just being a crossbreed is no guarantee of better health.

If your Cockapoo breeder claims that there is no need to do any health checks because the puppies benefit from hybrid vigor, it isn't true.

Ears and Skin

Spaniels are susceptible to both ear and skin problems and this is why the Cockapoo can suffer from these issues too. It's due to inheriting the Spaniels floppy ears (known as pendulous ears) which tend to trap moisture and dirt. Basically, their ears can trap bacteria and yeast, and because they are warm, it can lead to growth and spread. The most common ear condition is called Otitis which is inflammation of the ear canal and it's caused when the ear canal gets irritated by grass seeds, parasites, allergies or infections. It causes intense itching and you will notice your dog shaking her head, flapping her ears back and scratching them.

If you notice a smell, or you notice black or brown wax, or her ear looks red and she is scratching it then she may have an ear infection.

To help avoid this as much as possible you will need to check and clean your Cockapoo's ears regularly. Ask your veterinarian about appropriate ear care products then gently wipe out the ear with a cotton ball moistened with the cleaning solution that has been recommended. Avoid sticking the cotton swabs into her ear canal because that could damage it . If you are worried about how to clean her ears, then just ask your veterinarian to show you how best to clean them. I know that I have done that in the past.

To get her used to having her ears touched make sure you remember to touch and caress them when she is a puppy.

Like the ears, allergies can cause problems with the skin and they can lead to dermatitis (skin inflammation). They can be caused by many things including pollen or dust mites, items your dog eats (for example, wheat), items that your dog comes into contact with (for example, washing powders), or bites from parasites such as fleas.

As allergies cannot be cured, treatment might be needed for the rest of her life. But it is usually very effective and won't impact her other than requiring to have regular mediation. You will either be provided with special shampoo or you might need regular medication. I try to avoid steroids for long term use if I can but they can be effective in the short-term. There are a few other medications on the market that your vet might recommend.

Like Cocker Spaniels, Poodles are also prone to a variety of skin problems, including Sebaceous Adenitis. This causes dry, scaly skin with patches of hair loss on top of her head, and on the back of her neck, and back. This usually occurs when your dog is between one and five years of age. The condition usually requires a variety of long-term treatment and you may need to give fatty acid supplements and use special shampoos to remove dead skin and hair.

Eyes

If your Cockapoo is an F1 generation puppy from a Poodle father, then you should make sure the Poodle father has had a PRA test (Progressive Retinal Atrophy) but both Cockers and Poodles can suffer from this and it can lead to a loss of eyesight.

Cocker Spaniels can also suffer from a specific type of Glaucoma more than other breeds. This is known as Closed Angle Glaucoma. Ask your breeder if the Cocker parent has been screened recently for Glaucoma. Poodles also suffer from Glaucoma (Toy Poodles appear to be most prone to this). Symptoms include squinting, watery eyes, bluing of the cornea, and redness in the whites of the eyes and it is very painful.

If your puppy has redness in the white of her eyes your vet might test her for this disease.

More generally, you need to keep the hair around her eyes clean and short and you will need to trim around her eyes regularly.

Teeth

You will start getting your puppy used to having something in her mouth at an early age so that she will be comfortable with you cleaning her teeth when she gets older and needs it.

Use a dog tooth brush or, if you don't have one, then you can use a child's toothbrush. You should clean her teeth at last twice a week, and ideally every day. You can also use a dog dental chew. They love these, just don't overdo it - remember they are not treats.

Nails

Trim her nails once or twice a month. If you tend to walk on hard surfaces her nails will get worn down naturally and you may only need to get her nails checked or cut when she goes to the groomer. If you can hear them clicking on the floor, they might be too long.

Dog toenails have blood vessels in them, and if you cut too far you can cause bleeding so you might want to start by watching a groomer or asking for help from your veterinarian.

Coat And Grooming

Cockapoos are a good choice for allergy sufferers as they shed less than other breeds, but they do shed. Even although multi-generational breeding is often claimed to result in 'nonshedding' this is not the case. All dogs shed.

Cockapoo coats will vary, depending on their parentage. Their coats can range from straight due to their spaniel heritage (and type of spaniel) to wooly and curly from their Poodle heritage (and type of Poodle). Generally speaking they have wavy, long, fine hair that will need regular brushing to avoid becoming matted especially on their tummy's and legs. Their coats are usually white, cream, tan, brown or black in color.

The Cockapoo will benefit from professional grooming every 2-3 months and their coat should be two to three inches in length.

When you are grooming her, don't forget to check for any signs of infection such as redness, tenderness, or inflammation on the skin, eyes, and on her feet. This means that your weekly groom will help you spot any potential health problems early.

Dew claws

The first thing to point out is that dogs very rarely have dew claws in their hind legs - they are almost always only seen in the front legs - just above their pad and below the carpal pad. I tend to think about it as a thumb because it really is a thumb. While you can expect your Cockapoo to have two dewclaws, this is not the case for all breeds. The Great Pyrenees, for example, should have six dewclaws, one on each front leg and two on each hind leg and this is an AKC requirement.

When I was young, dew claws were removed from puppies when they were very young (anywhere between two and five days old) to 'conform to the breed standard'. It was also said that the dew claw might tear in later life and this would be very painful (it is). In those days, tails were docked at the same time depending on the breed requirements. I had the experience of being present during this process for all five of our first litter and it was not a pleasant experience. When dew claws are removed, the toe is severed off at the joint so that the entire toe is removed. It was, and still is, done without anaesthesia using an instrument that can only be described as a plier.

The practice of automatically removing dew claws in very young puppies is not as common these days - especially for Cockapoos. I no longer believe that they should be removed, and in later litters that I raised, we neither removed the dewclaws nor docked their tails. To this day I have never had a problem with one of my dogs' dew claws and have only recently known of a dog, a Cockapoo, who had a problem with her dew claw (she is 3 years old) and the conversation I had with her owner is worth including.

The dog, Poppy, had torn her dew claw while on a walk (she was being her usual self and darting and running about furiously through long grass) and was now on her way to the vets. This was not the first time this had happened, and the last time Poppy was taken into theatre in order to fix the dew claw, but not remove it. The question was - why did the vet simply cut the nail back and not remove the dew claw?

One of the reasons is that dew claws are attached to other tendons and muscles (and this is the case whether they are young puppies or older dogs, like Poppy). The front dew claws contain two bones. Attached to these bones are four tendons and two muscles. Once the dew claw is removed, these muscles are then left to atrophy, weakening the entire structure of the carpus and this can cause arthritis in the carpal.

The dew claws function is to stabilize the carpal joint when the dog is running or when she is making sharp turns. This stabilizing action gives additional traction and reduces the tension on the front leg. If a dog does not have its front dew claws, the leg will twist on its axis to overcompensate. This increases the pressure on the carpus and in turn, the rest of the forelimb all the way up to the shoulder.

A study published by the Journal of the American Veterinary Medical Association in 2018 looked at the risk factors for injuries in dogs involved with agility events. They concluded that the absence of the front dewclaws was one of the greatest factors "associated with significantly increased odds of injury". They went as far as to advise against the removal of the front dew claws from dogs being used in agility type activities.

Cockapoos can run around a lot, especially Poppy, and they need their dew claws to prevent further injury, rather than being the general of 'future' cause of injury. The argument to remove the dew claw 'incase of future injury' is, I believe, outweighed by the other, more serious and longer lasting injuries that we now know can be caused if a dog does not have its dew claw to help reduce the strain on other parts of her leg.

Loss of Blood/Weight

One of the first questions you should get asked by a veterinarian if you need to make an emergency call because your dog has had an injury is "is your dog bleeding". The reason they ask this is not because a dog can lose a lot of blood but that, even a small loss of blood, can be dangerous. Just two teaspoons per pound of weight can be enough to put your dog into shock. It is for this reason, if nothing else, that it is useful to always know the weight of your dog.

Von Willebrand Disease

This is a blood clotting disorder frequently found in Toy Poodles. Ask your breeder for the test for the Poddle parent - this is a DNA test.

Elbow and Hip Dysplasia

Cockapoos, although a small dog, are prone to hip and elbow dysplasia that usually progresses with age and may start to be visible when still a puppy. This disease, usually inherited from the Cocker Spaniel, is caused when the ball and sockets of the joint bones don't 'fit' properly and have a tendency to slip out. This causes the joint to form abnormally which can cause not only pain but mobility problems. Early signs can be a wobbly walk or your puppy lying with splayed back legs (best described as looking like a frog). If your puppy does this it might be nothing to do with dysplasia but if you are worried you can ask your veterinarian to test her for the disease. There are a number of treatments including medication, physiotherapy and even surgery.

Eating poop

I know another Cockapoo and at 10 weeks she was eating her poop. The owner called to ask what she should do.

It is not uncommon for a puppy to eat her poop - around 25% of them do it. Sometimes it is something they copied from watching their mother. When puppies are very young, and before they are weaned a mother eats her puppy's poop. This can continue during the early part of weaning. For us humans, it's quite hard to watch but it's perfectly natural for dogs. It is thought that it dates back to the days when they lived in the wild when the mother would need to keep the den clean and free from poop to protect the den from predators (and infections). For some puppies they will watch and learn this behavior but it usually doesn't last long.

Sometimes it's simply because puppies love taste and textures, and poop has both of these, plus it carries lots of interesting scents that has lots of information. Who the owner might be, what did they eat? And don't forget, puppies only have their mouths to explore with.

Research has found that dogs most likely to eat poop are hungry. If she is continuing to eat poop then make sure that you are feeding her at the correct intervals, and in the correct amounts and preferably to a schedule. You might also want to check that the food contains enough of the ingredients that she needs.

They can also eat poop because they are bored or stressed. Make sure she is not being left alone for too long and is getting plenty of stimulation. If you need to work, and are out of the house, try and get a dog sitter to visit.

Of all the reasons your puppy is eating poop the least likely is a nutritional deficiency in her diet. If she suddenly starts eating poop, especially if she is a bit older, then it might be due to a medical problem and in this instance you should contact your veterinarian.

To Spay or to Neuter your dog ?

Every Cockapoo owner is going to come up against this question but there really isn't any definitive right or wrong answer, either on the best timing or whether it needs to be done at all.

In the USA vets tend to recommend that pups are neutered or spayed as early as possible, usually around 8 weeks. In Europe and the UK most vets recommend 6–9 months and some recommend waiting until 10-24 months for males while females should be allowed to have at least two seasons.

It is now generally recommended that your dog has reached maturity before being spayed or neutered. This is because neutering and spaying removes hormones from your dog which have an important role to play in their development. These hormones regulate growth, mood, muscle, bone growth and density.

Some studies have shown an increased rate of, for example, Hip Dysplasia, in dogs that have had a neuter before maturity. If there is no medical reason to do it early, waiting until your dog reaches maturity might be better.

For female dogs, there are the added questions around whether it is beneficial to let the dog have a season before it is spayed. There is no evidence to show that having a season is in any way a healthy option for the dog, but the arguments about leaving a dog to reach maturity stand.

Here are some details of the pro's and con's but you should always check with your veterinarian.

Spaying

Spaying is the removal of the reproductive organs of the female dog and it can be either the removal of the uterus and ovaries or just the ovaries (which can be done using keyhole surgery). Removing both the uterus and the ovaries involves an abdominal operation and this is a bigger operation that requires an incision and needs a longer recovery time. It tends to be the most common operation. Regardless of the method the pro's and con's are the same.

The most obvious reason for spaying your dog is to avoid unwanted pregnancies closely followed by avoiding the regular seasons when she will be in heat. The medical benefits include reducing the risk of cancer in her reproductive organs and reducing the risk of Pyometra (which affects 23% of female dogs and leads to cysts in her uterus) and a reduced risk of peri-anal fistula (this is also known as anal furunculosis and more commonly affects German Shepherd Dogs). If it is done before she is 2.5 years old it can also reduce the risk of cancer in her mammaries .

Some of the arguments against spaying include the increased risk of urinary incontinence and increased urinary tract infections. It can also increase the risk of an under-active thyroid and increase the risk of obesity (in two spaniels that I know who were neutered later in life, both suffered significant weight gain). If the dogs are spayed before puberty there is a higher risk of vaginitis, and if done before 12 months (this timing will depend on the size of your dog) it can increase the risk of bone cancer.

Neutering

The operation for neutering your male dog is not as big as the female abdominal spay, The operation involves the removal of both testicles. After the operations it might look as if the dog still has his testes because the scrotal sac might initially retain the normal shape. It will usually shrink down over time.

One of the main reasons for neutering will be the desire to reduce the risk of your dog roaming in search of a female in season. We had a dog that did this and it was incredibly stressful. It made me think long and hard about what to do with Barney (he hasn't be spayed). The medical arguments for neutering include reducing the risks of testicular cancer and non cancerous prostate problems as well as reducing the risk of perineal fistula (again, more common with German Shepherd Dogs rather than Cockapoos).

The main arguments for not neutering include increasing the risk of hypothyroidism and obesity, and increasing the risk of prostate cancer. If it is done before he is 1 year of age there is an increased risk of bone cancer

For both sexes, the argument against neutering is the increased risk of an adverse reaction to vaccinations.

Finally, neutering will not fix behavioral problems including things like aggression and disobedience or resource guarding.

Chapter 3
Planning Ahead

Before you bring your puppy to her forever home, you need to find out what type of food your puppy has been eating up until this point. Your breeder will be happy to let you know and should provide you with a starter pack of what they have been feeding her. Don't worry if they don't do this as standard practice, just make sure that you know what you need to have in the house for your new puppy, and it needs to be what they have been eating up until this point.

You will introduce her to the food you want to use slowly. You will do this by mixing some of her existing food into the new food you have chosen, increasing the proportion of her new food gradually, over a period of 7-10 days. You also need to know how often she was being fed, and at what time she is used to being fed.

You need to do this because any sudden change to her diet will upset her tummy. It will make her feel uncomfortable and can result in unexpected accidents caused by diarrhoea that your puppy won't be in control of making it more difficult to successfully start potty training in these first few important days.

As you start to slowly change her food over you can also start to gradually change the time at which she gets her food so that the schedule moves to the times that works within your household.

Slowly changing to a new type of food by mixing the old with the new is a rule that you will follow throughout her life. Dogs - and their stomachs - don't like a sudden change to their diet. Always introduce a new dog food slowly, no matter how old your dog is.

Another important pre-coming-home requirement involves making sure that you have something that smells familiar to her when she arrives home. If the breeder doesn't have something you can take home with you, then ask if you can leave some clothing there for a week or so before you bring her home (a sock or an old towel).

Once she arrives home, put this item into the crate or basket that you want her to use. This will give your puppy some comfort over the first few days, and be a familiar smell for her and should help her settle in.

Finally, if you have a yard or garden, you will need to puppy-proof it. If there are any gaps in a fence or hedge, your puppy will find it, and she will disappear in a second to go exploring. You can use plastic chicken-wire or something similar but anything that will securely block access will do.

Remember to mix in some games with her potty and crate training. It's a great way to get the kids, and everyone else, involved in the care of your new puppy. This means that before your puppy arrives, work out who can do what and try and get all your household members involved as early as you can (this is also good for helping to prevent separation anxiety). You might want to try and get agreement to who does the morning, or lunch or evening or who's job it is to think up a game to play on a particular week or day.

And don't forget to pick the name of your puppy!

How to choose a name

Your puppy might already have a name, but if you are reading this before you have picked your puppy's name, then here are a few tips which can help you decide and that can make training easier.

Dogs hear at a higher frequency range than we do, and so choosing a name that ends with a vowel sound will help to grab her attention. Names that end in an 'ie ar 'ay' sound are best. Ideally, the name should start with a hard letter sound like B or D, and ideally, it should contain two syllables. For example Penny, Holly, Millie, Poppy, Rosie, Barney, Paddy.

But remember, you want to avoid any names that your puppy might confuse with one of your cues (like sit, stay, down, here or come).

Try and say the name a few times too because you need to make sure all the members of your family can say it - especially if they are toddlers - and that everyone is comfortable to shout the name in the park. My brother, for example, hated to shout the name Tootsie.

Although it's better to use her name from the very start, don't worry if you take a day or two to find just the right name that seems to fit your puppy's personality as you get to know her over these first few days. We once had a dog called Happy. It was her nickname when she was born because there was no better way to describe her, and we kept it because that's what she was. If you have a dog from a shelter, and you really want to change her name, or don't know what her name used to be, then give her a few days to get used to it (but it might take her a bit longer).

To get her used to her name, say it, and reward her when you say it even when there is no response. Then, as soon as there is a response, for example she looks in your direction, immediately reward her with a tastier treat. She is likely to be responding to the sound of your voice rather than her name but she will soon put two and two together. Just walk around the house and say her name and reward her response. Getting your puppy used to their name can be fun for us all.

Chapter 4
Welcome home
She's Arrived!

When your pup comes home, you will ideally already have her crate or basket ready. You will have the same type of dog food that she was being fed, and you will have the item placed in her crate or basket that smells familiar to her from her previous home.

Over the first few nights, she is likely to miss her old family. It is okay, over the first nights, to take her crate or basket into your room, but only do this for the first few nights.

She also won't be used to lots of noise and activity around her. Try and keep things as calm as possible, and make sure to create some 'time-outs' for her.

To introduce her to her crate, place it in the room where you tend to spend most of your time. If you have a room you want your puppy to stay in, then, after a day or two, move the crate into this room - but make sure you and the rest of the family spend time with her in that room.

And don't forget that puppies sleep a lot and they need their sleep. They will easily sleep for 7-8 hours at night, and they can sleep up to 14 hours a day. I will talk about a schedule later, and it will include sleep time for her.

But, in the early days, try to make sure that she gets her sleep time. Everyone will want to play with her. This is okay, and it's good for your puppy to have lots of affection because it will help her to get used to people and to being handled, but try and ensure that she gets a little break to get some sleep.

In terms of picking her up and cuddling her, try not to overdo her handling. Constantly picking her up will be something her little body is unlikely to be used to. Just like us, if we get picked up too much, it can become uncomfortable and even painful.

This isn't anything to worry about, but it's useful to be aware of how often she is being handled.

The best way to pick up your young puppy is to put your hands around her chest, then pull her towards your chest. As soon as she is safely secured, take one of your hands and use it to support her bottom so that you are supporting her weight - much like a baby.

Finally, don't forget to take a sniff of her breath! A puppy's breath has a unique smell, so grab your chance while you can! It disappears quickly!

Socialization

In its simplest form, socialization is how you and your puppy learn to communicate with each other and how your puppy learns about others that she lives with and meets. It is how she learns to live in her 'society' and interact with everything she meets including humans and dogs.

Having as many happy encounters as possible during her early weeks helps her to relate appropriately to humans of all ages, other dogs and to the situations that she will face day-to-day throughout her life.

Your puppy's first few weeks are really important for her socialization training, but this isn't easy in the first week or two because your puppy has yet to be vaccinated.

However, you can still carry her, take her out in your car, and have others come to the house to meet her. Try and let her meet as many adults and children as you can in the weeks before you can take her to classes. She should also meet other dogs at home if you know them, and you know that they are fully vaccinated.

This is also the best time to touch their ears, mouth, tails, and paws and to get her used to you doing this. This part of puppy training is often missed, but it will really help later with grooming, or if you need to inspect her for an injury.

Sit with her quietly so that you are also teaching her how to relax with you, and touch her ears or mouth, run your hand over her paws and her tail, and give her a treat and reward her when she remains calm and relaxed.

If you can, and as soon as you are allowed, and after her vaccinations allow it, take your puppy to socialization classes where she can meet other young puppies and their parents.

They will play around for 20 or 30 minutes, but they learn how to communicate with other dogs that they don't know and they learn how 'far they can go'. Dogs are pretty good at letting each other know when enough-is-enough! They also learn about meeting other humans who are not the family.

This part of her early training helps her feel comfortable with other dogs, she will learn what she can and can't do without getting a bark or, occasionally a nip, and she will be learning about meeting and interacting with other people.

Vaccinations over the first year

It's a good idea to talk to your vet about your puppy's vaccination requirements as soon as you can. Below is a summary of the recommended vaccinations from the American Kennel Club, and there are also optional vaccinations that you can give your puppy.

I have only included the recommended vaccinations here.

- 6-8 weeks - Distemper, parvovirus
- 10-12 weeks - DHPP (for distemper, adenovirus (hepatitis), parainfluenza, parvovirus
- 16-18 weeks DHPP, rabies
- 12-16 months DHPP, rabies

Unvaccinated puppies less than 4 months old are most at risk of Parvovirus.

Parvovirus is contagious and affects all dogs. There is no cure, and the puppy will need to be kept hydrated, and an effort made to control the secondary symptoms.

You can take her to your yard around 7 days after her first set of vaccinations, but avoid other dogs especially if you don't know them. Your yard must be enclosed to ensure no other dogs have been there. Her feet must not touch the ground in public spaces.

If you live in an apartment, you might need to go outside to a public or well-used street during her potty training and so that she can relieve herself. Pick one spot, and carry her there and back, and you can let her sniff around that spot.

After her second vaccination, you can take her for a walk on paved surfaces, but not on grass or places where you can't see if other dogs have urinated or gone to the toilet, although I would also suggest that you carry her, rather than walk her, on any surface.

It is still important for her not to meet unfamiliar dogs.

The Kennel Club recommends talking to your veterinarian about heartworm treatment when your puppy is 12-16 weeks old. This is a preventative medication that is taken regularly.

These are the sort of issues where any recommendation must come from a qualified pet health professional who understands the laws, and problems in your area, and who will be aware of any breed-specific problems. Make sure that you ask your veterinarian for advice.

Your puppy can go outside for a walk in the park after her third set of vaccinations (around weeks 16-18). It is also at this point that she can exercise for up to 20 minutes at a time.

She can now meet unfamiliar dogs and it is at this stage, when she is around 18 weeks, that you can take her to her puppy socialization classes at the local pet store or your vet (where all the other puppies will be at the same vaccination stage).

Chapter 5
House and Potty Training

O ne of the main reasons people don't want to have a puppy is the thought of potty training, or specifically, the thought of a dog that is not house-trained and that messes in the home.

House training or potty training your puppy will be one of the first things you do when your puppy comes home. It can be done, so don't worry. In fact, in the years to come you will forget that you ever had to house-train your beloved dog and won't even remember how you did it.

The speed at which a puppy learns will vary from puppy to puppy. How fast she learns can be helped by any training that had started in her previous home. I know this sounds obvious, but even a young puppy's rate of being house trained will depend on what they were taught once they were weaned and walking confidently on their 4 legs.

When we had a litter of 7 spaniels and we started to train the puppies to go to the puppy pad as soon as they reached the stage of moving around, which was around the time they were being weaned and as they moved on to solid food. It meant that when it was time to go to their forever homes they were much easier to potty train.

They were also familiar with using a cage. We kept it in the room with them so that they could wander in to play and sleep (and get used to its sound). It really can help a great deal.

How long can a puppy wait for the toilet

Don't forget that a puppy's bladder grows with them. So when they are younger, it is smaller, which means that they will need to empty it more often.

Generally speaking, a puppy's ability to hold its bladder increases by about an hour per month.

This will mean that at one month, they can hold on for about an hour. By 2 months old, they should be able to hold on for about 2 hours before they need to relieve themselves.

Try not to make them hold on for much more than this over the first few months, or there will be accidents, and try to make sure that your time away from them can tie into their need to go to the toilet.

As a general rule, puppies under 6 months will struggle to hold their bladder for more than 3 or 4 hours, and this should help you work out how long you can be away or when you might need to try and get someone to visit your puppy so that they can relieve themselves outside, rather than in their crate, or in the room they are in.

In terms of pooping, a puppy will poop after food. If you feed your puppy before you leave, make sure that you feed them around 45 minutes before you are due to leave.

This gives you time to take them for a poop. They will normally need to poop between 5 and 30 minutes after a meal. Millie poops about 5 minutes after her meal, while Barney is about 20 minutes.

If you are playing with your puppy before you leave, take them out for a poop after the playtime, as this can also make them want to poop.

Puppy Pads

The best thing I have used for potty training is puppy pads and the very best thing I ever tried was a puppy pad that looked like grass. For some reason, it really works. I used it with the seven puppies before they left for their forever homes, and they all used it. They would actually go to it without any prompting.

Whether you use a fabric pad or a fake grass one, these are the things you need to do.

I started by placing the puppy pad in the room as soon as my puppy, Millie, came home. Then, when she looked like she was about to potty, I would place her on the pad, and if she relieved herself, she got lots of praise. It didn't take long - probably around 2-3 days - before she would go to the pad.

I then started to move the puppy pad towards the door that I wanted her to use to go out. Try not to move it too far from where you started the training; just move it slowly to that door.

Once at the door, I let her get used to that for a day or two then I moved the pad just outside the back door.

In the final stages, if I saw her starting to pee or potty in the house, I would gently pick her up and place her an 'emergency' pad, and then I would take her and the pad outside. If there was not enough time to do this, I would just place her on the pad.

You might want to consider placing the puppy pad at the door that she will be using to access her outside area right away. Of course, this will depend on how far from the room the household congregates is from that door. You don't want to place it too far from where she will be spending most of her time in these early days.

At every point, every little win, give your puppy lots of praise.

This process can take more time for some puppy's than for others. However, as long as you remember that she will want to relieve herself when she wakes up, after play, and after she eats, then you have a head-start knowing when to expect activity. Make sure you take her outside after each of these events - don't only rely on the puppy pad.

It's important never to punish or get angry with your puppy if she toilets in the house. You sometimes see a recommendation to push their face into the mess. Don't do this. It will do the opposite of helping. They won't understand and will be scared. Getting angry or pushing them may only mean that they don't want to potty in front of you and learn to avoid it.

How to manage their potty training

Puppy's (and later dogs) love praise and rewards.

Once your puppy begins the process of going outside to potty, don't forget that every time she relieves herself outdoors, you need to praise her and give her a treat.

Don't do this while she is in the action of potty-time - she will stop to seek the reward, get distracted, and won't finish what she started, which means that she won't be fully relieved when she goes back inside. Instead, wait until she has finished, and don't forget to do this every single time she goes outdoors to potty.

As you do this, use a phrase that she will start to recognize (try not to use 'Good boy' or 'Good girl' - it might cause confusion!). I used to say 'Be a good girl' and, on reflection, this wasn't a great idea.

Instead, use a short phrase such as 'potty' or 'pee pee' or whatever you feel comfortable saying and will remember - just make sure it is one that your pup can begin to recognize with the action she is being asked to complete. This is a key step because they need to know exactly what behavior the reward is for.

This is not only useful when your puppy is young. Millie, my older dog, had soft tissue damage to her knee on her hind leg. This meant that she struggled to walk and had difficulty 'sitting down' to toilet.

When I carried her to the garden to try and get her to 'do pee-pee,' this was much easier because I could say a phrase, and she knew exactly what I wanted her to do and she wanted to make me happy. It's good to remember that much of what you teach now will be of great help throughout your dog"s life. It's also good to think about what phrase you will be stuck with for a long time!

In her early days you will be tempted to take her into the yard every hour to play with her - try not to overdo the this. Stick to around 15 minutes at a time. And don't confuse her by taking her out to play when you want her to potty. I had someone do this with their puppy and they couldn't understand why she did not potty outside but kept doing it inside. The problem was that the puppy thought outside was only for play and didn't know what was expected of her. The puppy had lots and lots of fun but his mum was getting no work done and getting more and more frustrated. Try and set a clear distinction between when you are taking her out to potty and when you are taking her out to play. The schedule will help plan this and help train you to do both potty and play.

Where?

Choose a place or a small area outside where you want her to relieve herself. As she relieves herself, say your word or specific phrase.

Always take her to the same place every time you take her out to potty - in the morning, the last thing at night, after food, or after play during the day.

If you are using training pads overnight, take the soiled pad to the outside area where you want your puppy to toilet. The scent can help her.

When it is time to take her outside to toilet, avoid playing with her and getting her excited before she relieves herself. Remember, she is easily distracted and will forget what she is there to do.

If your puppy looks a bit confused or doesn't toilet right away, try to encourage her to sniff the ground beside the area you want her to use.

Stay outside with her until she toilettes. If nothing happens after 5 minutes, don't start to play with her but take her back inside but watch her closely.

After 10 minutes, take her out again and repeat the process until she has done what you need her to do.

The signs to watch out for

Try and supervise your puppy at all times when you are trying to potty train her. I know this is very hard to do, but by supervising and watching her, you will notice how she looks when she starts to feel uncomfortable because her bladder is full, and you will start to recognize how she reacts when this happens.

For example, she might start circling or sniffing the floor, she might be restless, and she may try and go to a place where she has previously done her business.

If you see your puppy mid-toilet, pick her up and take her outside and try to get her to finish what she started there; if she does, then gently praise her.

Now, this is hard to describe, and it's not something that is often described, but watch your puppy's bottom.

When they need to go poop, you will notice their rear end swelling outwards. This means a poop is imminent. To this day, I watch Millie and Barney's rear ends when we are out walking (usually it's the start of a walk), and I get the poop bags ready.

As you will have learned already, puppies and dogs are all a bit different in how they prefer to poop and pee.

When Millie was a puppy, she was obviously getting restless and looking around for a place to pee-pee but when Barney was young, he was really difficult to read because he didn't do any obvious things like scratching at the door, sniffing, or circling he just 'looked a certain way' and was restless in a different way that he usually was.

Watch out for any of those signs, or watch out for something your dog does that might signal a change in behavior. This is the part where they train us. We need to watch and learn what they are telling us.

I would, though, also recommend keeping them to just one or two rooms as you go through the house-training process—be vigilant; watch, learn, and stay with them if you can,

Leaving the house and overnight

It is possible that your puppy won't be able to hold her bladder all night long for several months. This means that she will need to relieve herself during the night.

Put some newspaper or puppy pads in her crate. Try and place them in an area that she can avoid. In the morning, don't forget to remove the soiled pad or newspaper and then take it to her outside area to try and draw her to the scent.

If you are going out for any length of time, and you are using her crate, then you will do the same thing. If you can, don't be away for more than 2-3 hours at the start.

It may take several months before your puppy is fully house trained, but the accidents will become less frequent. Try and be patient. It will pay off in time, and in just a few short years, you will have forgotten all about the trials and tribulations of potty training your puppy.

How to clean up

It's important to clean the area and try to remove the scent.

Don't use ammonia-based products as this will just encourage them to go to the same place again. I have found that cold water can do the trick, too (and it is very good at removing any staining). You can use biological powder, and some people swear by a vinegar-water mix. I have tried this, but I am not convinced it works, although I know other dog owners where this has worked wonders.

Your schedule

One of the best and most effective ways to train your puppy is to get her used to a schedule.

When you first bring your puppy home, make sure that you take her out frequently. Take her out as soon as she wakes up, after playing, and after she has eaten or had a drink.

4 step summary of a puppy schedule:-

1. Feed them at the same time and the same frequency, for example, every 2 hours depending on their age
2. Take them out them out as soon as they wake up
3. Take them out before they go to bed
4. Take them out after food and after indoor puppy play.

In terms of how a day might look, try not to forget her sleep time. Your puppy will get sleepy after eating but make sure that you take her out to potty before she goes for her nap.

I tend to let my dogs out as soon as they wake up. I then feed them breakfast and play with them for 20-30 minutes (depending on how much time I have), then I take them out again before they fall asleep. They have been doing this schedule since they were young pups, and they seem to like it. These days, as adults, Barney will potty as soon as he wakes up but Millie is more interested in breakfast and so will wait until after she has been fed. They will both urinate as soon as they wake up and before breakfast.

Finally, once she is older don't feed her right before you take her out for a walk and don't feed her as soon as you return from a walk. The reason you do this is to avoid something called GDV (Gastric Dilatation-Volvulus).

GDV is often known as dog bloat, or a twisted stomach, gastric or gut. It is caused by a number of things including large meals, stress, anxiety, excitement and vigorous exercise. It tends to be more common in larger dogs such as German Shepherds but it is worth bearing in mind for Cockapoos because many will eat their food extremely fast. This can impact the potential for GDV. If they are very fast easters you can reduce the amount they get fed in one sitting, and compensate by more frequent feeding.

GDV usually occurs within the first two hours of eating, and so the general rule has been to wait 30 minutes after feeding before taking them for a walk and to wait 30 minutes after a walk before feeding them (a gap between exercise and food of 30 minutes). Some vets will recommend waiting for at least two hours after eating before you exercise them and to wait 30 minutes after exercise before feeding.

Sleep

As mentioned earlier, puppies sleep a lot. When she is young and up to 3 months old, she can sleep 18 hours a day, sometimes up to 20!

She can fall asleep suddenly, and it can even appear as if she has fallen asleep mid-step. She will fall asleep with a chew in her mouth or just sit down in the middle of the floor and collapse. When she does, just pick her up and put her in her crate or basket (with the door open).

She should easily sleep for 7 hours at night, and some puppies can sleep for 7 hours without requiring a bathroom break.

Puppies need their sleep, so make sure you don't forget to let her get it. This will be harder than you think in the first few weeks. There will be many visitors and lots of people who will want to pick her up and cuddle her. This is okay but don't forget to give her sleep time. She needs it.

Build this into your schedule so that it might look like this:

7:15 am - wake up and go outside for potty
7:30 am - breakfast
8:00 am - playtime
8:15 am - outside for toilet
8:20 am - sleep (with toy in the cage/depart for work?)
10:15 am - outside for toilet
10:30 - food
10:35 - outside for toilet
11:00 - playtime
11:15 - outside for toilet
11:20 am - sleep with Kong or Toy in the cage
1:15pm - wake up/ outside for toilet
1:20pm - food
1:25 - outside for toilet
2:00 - playtime
2:15 pm - outside for toilet
2:20 - sleep (cage with toy)

And so on. You will find a schedule that works for you as you discover when your puppy likes to go potty during the day. It might be after food or after playtime. But always take her out as soon as she awakens.

These timings will change as she gets a bit older and sleeps less —but she will always sleep a great deal, some Cockapoos can sleep up to 14 hours a day although this is not the norm.

Note that the schedule separates playtime from toilet time. I have mentioned this earlier in the book. You are aiming to distinguish between potty time and playtime.

In her younger days playtime will usually be indoors but you will want to play with her outside too, if you have a yard. You will need to try and make a distinction between going out to play and going out to potty because she will need to know what it is that you expect her to do when you take her outside.

Don't think that taking her outside alone will indicate that she should try to go to the toilet so don't take her outside to play and at the same time expect her to know that a part of that play-time is toilet time. She will simply be ready to play every time she goes outside.

You should aim to separate the activity in each outside visit when you are potty training her. You could, for example, wait until she potties before any play can start. After she potties and gets her praise and reward you can calmly wait for a minute and then signal the start of playtime. Try and mix playtime inside and out over the first few weeks so that she gets the hang of an outside visit being for potty time.

Bedtime

You will find that your puppy will start to go to bed by herself as she gets used to your schedule, and she will soon fit in with your own bedtime.

In the early days, if she does wake up during the night, don't make a fuss and do not be tempted to play with her. She will be more than happy to play, but she needs to learn that this is not the right time. Don't turn on all the lights or it will seem like daytime to her. Take her outside to let her toilet and then return her to her bed.

Dogs should always have access to water but during her potty training at night time you may decide to remove her water bowl. Do this no more than 2 hours before she goes to bed, and make sure that she has had a recent drink first, she needs her water. This will help keep her bladder less active during the night.

Chapter 6
Crate Training

Many people worry that using a crate might be cruel. If used properly, a crate is a place where your puppy will feel safe and happy - it will be her den. The main objective of your crate training is to teach her that the crate is her 'safe place' and that it belongs to her. Never use her crate as a 'sin bin'.

Using a crate will also bring with it a range of other benefits that will mean your life with your puppy can be as full and as engaging as possible - and it will allow her to be included in almost all of your activities, including vacations or holidays. Crate training is often one of the best ways to help speed up house training.

The reason using the crate works for house training is that dogs don't like to mess where they sleep, and where they relax. Your puppy will not mess here, especially if you have crate trained her to view her crate as her safe place. What's more, if she is sleeping in her crate, she will do her very best to hold on until she can leave her crate.

This puts you in more control, because you will know where your puppy is, and what she might want to do when you open the door, or when she leaves her crate, especially if she has been sleeping in her crate. Remember, you will always take her outside to toilet as soon as she wakes up and it is a good idea to do this every time she leaves the crate if she has been in there for 30 minutes or more, even if she has not been sleeping.

Crate training has lots of other benefits and your dog will be able to travel with you more easily. You can visit friends and family more easily because you can use the crate as her portable bed. It also means that you can go out knowing that you won't return to chewed furniture or a general mess (the chewing usually only occurs with puppies), and your dog can use the crate as her bed during the day and during the night.

In summary, the crate gives your dog and puppy somewhere safe to rest and to sleep. It helps her feel comfortable when you leave the house; she can feel safe in a new house or room that you are visiting, and it means that she can enjoy more of your life outside of the home if you need to travel.

It will also help her settle with a dog sitter or if she needs to go and stay away from home when you go on vacation.

Introducing your puppy to the crate

After picking your crate, and before she arrives home, add a blanket or something soft for your puppy to lie on. Ideally add an item that has a familiar scent for her.

If you are using a second-hand crate, make sure you wash it thoroughly to remove any scent from the previous dog who may have been using it.

If you are using a wire crate, have something like a sheet or a blanket that you can place on top of it as well as around the sides. Don't cover up all four sides, and make sure the front of the crate (where the door is) is left uncovered. This can help to make it feel more like a den, especially at night.

Initially, you can place the crate in a room that is used by the rest of the household. This will help the puppy get used to the crate without being separated from you and the rest of the family, and it will mean she doesn't feel alone and scared. A puppy will not be used to being alone, and it will make her anxious and scared, especially when she first arrives home. Having company around her will be important.

If you want to, you can put the crate into the room that you want her to use and then follow the steps below. Once you pick your room make sure that you also spend lots of time there with her.

When your puppy comes home, place her toys, and, if you have not already done so, add the scented item from her previous home, into the crate.

The first stage is to place some food around the crate. If she doesn't start moving towards the crate, or being curious about it all by herself, then entice her by calling her to the crate in a happy tone of voice, and by throwing tasty treats around and near the crate. Keep trying until she starts to come over to the crate and begins to feel comfortable around it.

The second stage is to slowly start moving the treats to the door, and then inside the crate. Give her lots of praise at all stages. Only start moving the treats inside the crate once she has started getting used to the outside of the crate. As she starts to enter the crate, don't close the door.

Keep playing the game and move the treats deeper into the crate. Just let her enter and leave and explore if she wants to. You want to get her used to entering and leaving by herself.

It can take anything from 10 minutes to a few days, depending on her experience to date, to get her to go into her crate by herself. Keep the training sessions to between three and five minutes.

If, for any reason, your puppy is not responding to food or treats, then entice her with her favorite toy (some dog breeds prefer toys to treats but Cockapoos usually favor a treat).

The third stage is to increase the length of time she spends in her crate. You can do this by feeding her in her crate, or you can put a Kong toy filled with treats into the cage, for her to play with.

If she is reluctant to go into the crate, put her food bowl beside the crate door, and then slowly move it into the crate until she eats at the back of the crate.

Once she is happy entering and leaving and lingering for a few minutes in her crate, try to close the door. You can do this when she is eating, but one of the most effective ways is to give her the Kong stuffed with something she loves.

Wait until she starts to become engrossed in getting her food out of the Kong, then slowly close the door. If you close the door and she gets anxious or scared, immediately open the door.

If she does nothing, then wait for a few minutes before opening the door again.

Keep increasing the length of time before you open the door. You are aiming to reach 10 minutes. If she shows any signs of distress, if she is panting, whining, cowering, or showing any signs of aggression, then you will know you have increased the time too quickly.

Once your puppy is happy to stay in the crate for up to 10 minutes after eating or playing, then you will know that she is now likely to understand that this crate is her safe space.

The last stage of her crate training can now begin, and this is when you move out of sight, while she is in her crate with the door closed.

This is the stage when her toys and her Kong (filled with food, peanut butter, or soft cheese) will really help.

Put her toys in her crate, and close the door once she has entered. Stay beside the crate for around five minutes before moving quietly from the room and out of sight.

Once you are out of sight, turn around and come back to the side of the crate and sit beside it for 5 minutes. Gradually start to stay out of sight longer. Do this throughout the day but at different times. You will need to repeat the process several times.

If you hear any barking or whining, do not come back mid bark or mid whine. Try and find a gap, and this is when you return. You are aiming to increase the time you are out of sight to around 30 minutes.

Once this has been achieved, you can start leaving the house altogether. But remember to provide toys for her to play with, so that she does not get bored. Before leaving, make sure she has had a small meal and has been exercised, and remember to leave calmly without any fuss.

In terms of sleeping at night, you can put the crate in your bedroom at night in the early days. You only want to do this for a few days and not any longer.

When your puppy first arrives home, she will have been used to sleeping with other puppies, so letting her sleep in her crate in your room will help her settle in.

Once you put the crate into the room where she will normally spend her night, make sure to turn out the lights when you (and she) go to bed. You can leave a low-level one on if you like, but make sure it isn't bright.

This will also mean that if you need to take her out during the night, she will recognize that this is sleep time. And don't forget that if you need to take her out during the night, don't turn on all the lights.

Size and Types of Crate

There are 3 main types of crate. A plastic crate (or box), a wire crate or cage, and one made of fabric. I use the fabric case as a travel carry case and use it as a den when we are staying away from home overnight.

I use both a cage (in the house) and a fabric crate for travel, but I know many people who use a plastic crate. The choice is up to you.

What size?

Unlike the crate's material, the size of the crate that you choose is important.

If the crate is too small, it will make your dog uncomfortable, and if it is too big, it can make your dog insecure. You need to know the height, width, and length of the crate.

The crate size will depend on both the weight and height of your puppy when she is fully grown. Because Cockapoos can come from different sizes of both Cocker Spaniel and Poodle, as well as a first or second generation of Cockapoo, sizes can vary. The table below gives a general size and weight guide.

Finally, to save you from buying different crates as your puppy grows, you can section off a part of the crate with a separator to make it smaller when she is smaller.

The recommended Cockapoo crate size is usually 30" and this allows for dogs weighing up to 40lbs and between 18"-19" in height. If you have a Maxi you might want to check the height of her parents.

The table of Cockapoo height and weight is added again here to save you going back to the start of the book.

	Standard/ Maxi	Miniature	Toy	Teacup
Height	16 – 22 inches	11 – 15 inches	10 – 11 inches	Under 10 inches
Weight	Over 25 lbs	13 – 25 lbs	6 – 12 lbs	Under 6 lbs
Age when full grown	12 – 14 months	9 – 12 months	7 – 9 months	5 – 7 months

Cockapoo Height and Weight Range

Chapter 7
Food and Feeding

As we have discussed earlier, you need to get your puppy into a regular schedule. The quicker you can do this and get her used to this schedule, the easier everything becomes. Creating a schedule really can make a big difference.

Feeding them to the same schedule also means that they will want to relieve themselves in reaction to that schedule. This, in itself, will make it easier for you to house-train.

What to feed them

Dogs are built to be meat-eaters, but they are descended from omnivores, so they can survive adequately without meat (if the protein balance is right).

The protein in meat is not the same as the protein found in plant-based foods, and this is one of the reasons to be careful of the food you give your puppy and your dog.

This doesn't mean that dogs can't live on a plant-based diet; it just means it will need to be supplemented with the essential proteins that she will require as well as Vitamin D.

Balancing nutrition is the most important aspect of your dogs' food. For example, we need our carbs for energy, but dogs don't need many carbs.

Dogs, and especially puppies, need fats and fatty acids. Most of these are contained in animal fats, but some seed and plant oils can provide a concentrated source of energy. You are looking for an Omega-3 family of essential fatty acids.

When looking for dog food, look at the type of calories rather than the overall total. For example, you don't want too much carbohydrate.

Today's average dog food can contain anywhere between 30% and 70% carbohydrates, but in the wild, dogs will intake only about 15%.

An adult dog's diet can contain up to 50% carbohydrate (by weight), up to 4.5% fibre, and a minimum of around 5.5% should come from fats, and 10% from protein.

You can read more about nutrition at nap.edu, and this is listed in the resources at the end of this book.

In general, though, if you want to check out how much meat is in your dog food, look at the ingredients list. The further down the meat appears, the lower the meat content.

The most common ingredients today are whole grain, fat, soya, and corn. So if you see chicken by-products, this doesn't mean it is chicken meat. It most likely isn't.

The top ingredients to look for (and look for a range of these in the same food) include deboned chicken or turkey, Atlantic mackerel and herring, chicken and turkey liver, chicken and turkey heart, and other items such as egg and other types of fish. All high in protein.

There has also been some debate about dry food versus wet food. The main difference being that wet food contains more water (around 75%) whereas dry food can contain only about 10% water.

Dry food tends to be more calorie-dense, and wet food has less grain and fewer carbs. Grain isn't necessarily a bad thing, it just depends on quantity.

Dry food lasts for longer and tend to be more cost-effective than wet food.

There are lots of choices on the market, and you will want to research this for yourself. I feed Millie and Barney wheat-free dry fish-based kibble, but I try to change this from time to time. I have now found a brand that they love that comes from a local farm producer.

Sometimes, I mix in some wet food. They really love this, and I quite like the mix of wet and dry food as a balance. It's important to vary their food and its texture from time-to-time to give them a little change. Like many smaller dogs, Cockapoos can be fussy eaters so varying their diet (and sometimes portion size) can keep them engaged and interested in their food. You may also discover something that they love and decide to stick with it.

Some owners also like to feed their dog a raw diet known as RAW or a BARF diet (Bones and Raw Food). There are quite a few sites online that can explain how to do this and what this diet includes. A key to this diet is balance and The Natural Dog site (A Guide to Raw Diet and Health The Natural Way) is a good place to start if this is something that you are interested in finding more about.

How much to feed

Puppies can require up to double the energy intake of adult dogs. This is based on the weight of your puppy - it doesn't mean they eat twice as much as an adult dog, just that per pound of weight they do.

Depending on your type of Cockapoo, they will reach their adult weight anywhere between 5 and 14 months old. You can check the table in Chapter 1 or at the end of the last chapter for the expected size and weight which includes the average time until they reach their adult weight.

Although Cockapoos can be fussy eaters they also love to eat - probably as a result of their constant energy - which is also also a typical trait of Cockers. This means that it is best to control their feeding and not leave food in their bowl for them to nibble on between meals.

The frequency really does depend on how old they are. A puppy's tummy is small and it grows over time. This means that you need to feed smaller amounts more regularly, the younger they are.

Puppies aged 8-16 weeks need to be fed 4 meals a day, perhaps every 3 hours. Pups ages 3 to 6 months should be fed 3 times a day (every 4 hours) and then after that twice a day, in the morning and early evening.

Your aim is to spread their nutrition throughout the day, so space out the times to equal intervals across the day. Once you are taking your puppy out for walks, which will mean more exercise, remember not to feed your puppy just before or after exercise.

The amount that you feed your puppy will depend on their weight and age. The dog food you choose will also have a variety of different protein levels.

When you decide on your dog food, the packaging will tell you how much to feed your puppy (depending on their weight). If you are in any doubt, ask your veterinarian.

What not to feed - dangerous foods for your dog

Alcohol - under no circumstances give your dog alcohol. In the worst-case scenario, alcohol can cause death.

Caffeine and chocolate—don't give your puppy anything with caffeine. Things that can include caffeine are obviously coffee, but chocolate can also contain caffeine. Chocolate, especially dark chocolate, should never be given to your dog. The toxic substances can cause vomiting, irregular heart function, and even death. If your dog has eaten a lot of chocolate, contact your veterinarian immediately.

Coconut (including coconut oil) - might cause stomach upsets, but coconut water should not be given to your dog.

Onion, chives, and **garlic** can irritate the bowel and are toxic to dogs.

Nuts (Pecans, Almonds, Walnuts, Macadamia) - these have the potential to not only cause vomiting but possible pancreatitis.

Raisins and grapes - avoid giving your dog raisins or grapes. The effect the toxins have is still not definitive, but it can cause Kidney failure. This also includes other dried variants like sultanas and currants and any foods containing grape, such as grape juice, raisin cereal, raisin bread, granola, trail mix, and raisin cookies or bars. Early signs are vomiting, diarrhea, and lethargy.

Raw Potato (or green potato) is poisonous to dogs. It contains a toxic compound called solanine (which is also contained in green tomato's), and if your dog eats a large amount, it will affect his nervous system. Symptoms to look for are blurred vision, vomiting, diarrhea, low temperature, and slow heart rate.

Bones - Generally speaking, be careful of any bones that you give your dog to chew. Avoid cooked bones because they tend to splinter and they can puncture their digestive tract if they swallow these splinters. If they can easily break a bone apart (raw or cooked), they can lodge in their throats or their intestines. They love bones so just pick your bone carefully.

Shellfish - some dogs are okay with shellfish, but one of my dogs will vomit immediately, and this will happen with even small traces of shellfish such as prawns or langoustine. This doesn't mean dogs can't eat fish. They can eat fish, and fish is good for them in many cases. Always ensure it is cooked and sufficiently cooled.

Xylitol (sweetener) and all foods containing Xylitol is toxic to dogs. It can cause your dog's blood sugar to drop and cause acute liver failure and even death. Early symptoms include vomiting, lethargy, and coordination problems or seizures. Xylitol is used as a sweetener in several products including candy, gum, baked goods, diet foods, and even some peanut butter and toothpaste.

What to do if your pet is poisoned

These are the instructions from the Pet Poison helpline:-

- Remove your pet from the area.
- Check to make sure your pet is safe: breathing and acting normally.
- Do NOT give any home antidotes.
- Do NOT induce vomiting without consulting a vet or Pet Poison helpline.
- Call Your Vet or, in the US, the Pet Poison helpline. The number is 855-764-7661.
- If veterinary attention is necessary, contact your veterinarian or emergency veterinary clinic immediately.

Bear in mind that it is always better when a toxicity is reported immediately, so don't wait to see if your dog becomes symptomatic before calling for help. There is a narrow window of time when your puppy can be decontaminated (induced vomiting or pumping the stomach) in the case of a poisoning.

Chapter 8
Chewing and Mouthing

P uppies not only chew but there is a period when they will use their mouths - a lot! This is called mouthing, and their tiny teeth are remarkably sharp.

They will grab your trouser legs or put their mouth around your hands - and their sharp teeth will take your breath away.

Puppies need to learn about different textures - and human skin is just one of the textures they need to learn about. They also need to understand how hard they can close their jaws, and when enough is enough. They can only learn this by doing it. If you have children then you need to be very aware of this.

Mouthing

All puppies will go through this phase, and you will want to teach them about 'bite inhibition'.

This is something that puppies, who have come from a larger litter, will have learned a bit about, because they usually learn this through play with other puppies (and something early socialization classes can help too).

There were many times when Millie had her brood of seven puppies, that we heard squeals of outrage or pain, as they pushed each other over and mouthed at ears, paws, and anything they could get their mouths around.

When one of the pups squealed, they would stop playing, but so did the protagonist. That pup tended to look as surprised as the pup that got a sharp tooth implanted into it. Yet, just a few moments later, they were back playing.

It was notable that the pup that got the painful nip was pretty eager to try this out on one of the other unsuspecting puppies.

This is just a part-and-parcel of a puppy growing up and learning boundaries. But it doesn't make it easier or any less painful. However, over time, all seven of the puppies seemed to understand each other and know how hard a bite they could get away with. The screams of surprise between them became less frequent.

Puppies are most likely to try and mouth you when you are playing with them, tickling their tummy, or petting them.

Nor surprisingly, the best way to deal with mouthing is to behave like a puppy.

First of all - it's important to let your puppy mouth you.

Let her have your hand. When she closes her mouth too hard, and her sharp teeth become painful, squeal like a puppy or use the word "stop" and then stop playing with her. Just let your hand go limp so that it is no fun to play with.

This should stop your puppy for a moment or two. She will be just as surprised as you. When she relaxes her mouth and stops, then praise her. Then let her have your hand again.

She will definitely go too far quite a few times, so just keep repeating over a 15- or 20-minute time intervals until she learns how hard she can close her mouth without hurting you.

If your squealing and "stop' doesn't work, then put her on the "naughty step' so to speak. Stop playing with her for 30 seconds or so. After this, start playing with her again.

If she does it again, then repeat, and if this still doesn't work, then move away from her as soon as she mouths you and you feel that nip.

As the hard biting stops, you will want to continue teaching her as she moves her mouthing levels down from sore to moderate. Slowly teaching her not to mouth at all.

Eventually, she will know exactly the level of pressure that she can safely apply when she is playing.

Whatever you do, don't hit your puppy for mouthing. This will only make her play harder, but it may also cause her to fear you.

Remember not to jerk your hands away from your puppy when she starts mouthing you. She still thinks this is a game and is more likely to lunge forward. Likewise, don't wave your hands in front of her face for the same reason - she will think that this is a game too.

Once you have done this, you want her to learn not to mouth at all on human skin, and to let you pet her without being mouthed.

When your puppy tries to mouth you when you are petting them, distract her by giving her a treat or a chew toy. I ended up using a tug toy with Millie. I waved it in front of her and just said, "Play Tug."

This worked really well because she used to follow me around and grab my ankles to get me to play with her. To stop her doing this I would stand still and say, "play tug." It's classic distraction training!

When she stopped trying to grab my ankles, I would praise her. Eventually, I could walk around without being tailed by a puppy with sharp teeth.

One last thing to bear in mind. Like all toddlers, puppies can have tantrums. I know a Cockapoo who really likes her tantrums! Her body will be stiffer, and her mouth might be tighter around the lips.

If you notice this while you are playing with her, just stop the play.

Don't squeal if she bites you (it will be harder than normal). If you are holding her, stop playing but continue to hold her for a few seconds, then let her go.

Don't make her afraid of you, uou just want her to know that she has gone too far. If you notice that your puppy continues to have tantrums, you will need to get more help from a professional.

Chewing

Most dogs like to chew, and some breeds are more likely to chew than others. For example, Labradors and Staffordshire Bull Terriers tend to have a stronger desire to chew. Because

Cockapoos are intelligent with moderate energy, they need a lot of mental stimulation and if they are bored, they will be inclined to chew.

All puppies enjoy and need to chew. They do this to explore their environment and understand the texture of things; they don't have hands, and they like to pick things up. So the only way that she can explore is to use her mouth.

All puppies go through the teething phase which also causes chewing. Depending on your type of Cockapoo, she will start to experience discomfort in her mouth as her teething process gets underway anywhere between three and seven months. She will chew to help remove her baby teeth, and she will chew to help with the pain of her adult teeth erupting in her gums.

As your puppy starts to reach adolescence, her chewing is going to get worse. There are two possible reasons for this.

It is around now that she will tend to get easily bored so try to find new games (especially mental exercise games) and other games to keep her occupied.

It is also around this time that her adult teeth are settling into the jaw, which can be uncomfortable for some dogs.

Whatever the reason, and it might be both of the above reasons, your puppy is going to chew at things.

In my case, it was furniture. This included the legs of tables, the sides of the sofa, shoes, wallets, and spectacles.

You will need to teach everyone in your household to put their shoes out of reach, and preferably out of sight, along with any toys that have different textures. These will be the favored chew items. Puppies love shoes - they are just about the right consistency of hard and soft making them perfect for exploring different textures. Much the same as furniture too.

Don't forget that your puppy might chew all of her life (mine stick to tennis balls now), but it will never be as bad as that first year. Dogs chew when they get older because it relaxes them and it's a calming activity (and they enjoy it).

Here are some chew toys and tips that might help.

- Try and change your dog's chew toys regularly by rotating them every few days. This will prevent her from getting bored and prevent her from looking for something else to chew that might look more interesting.
- Remove anything that you don't want her to chew and keep everything well out of reach. I lost a TV remote control and a pair of glasses by forgetting to move them to higher ground.
- If you find your puppy chewing on something that is not allowed, don't punish her or shout at her. This will only make her anxious. Instead, simply distract her attention and then direct her to a chew toy that you want her to play with. When she starts to play with it, make a fuss of her.
- Don't forget to remove anything dangerous to your puppy when she cannot be supervised. This includes some types of household plants (see below for some examples) that are poisonous to dogs. And watch out for wires that run along the floor.
- Many hard plastic toys are not made for chewing by a dog. The best chew toys are made of the type of hard rubber that you get with your Kong. You can also consider activity balls (like Kong's, you can place

kibble, cheese spread, peanut butter, or other treats or food inside). Ropes are also good but avoid nylon or anything that she can pull apart into a string.

- Chews such as dental chews or other edible chews can distract your puppy - but they can be eaten quite quickly. These chews last just a few minutes with Barney, so I tend to use them less as a chew alternative. Some dogs can chew for quite some time on these, though. It is just a case of testing which chews your puppy likes the most.

- Keep all house plants well out of reach, especially the ones that are poisonous to dogs. Here are a few examples: Cyclamen, Poinsettia, some Lilly's, Oleander, Brunfelsia, Aloe, Amaryllis (bulbs), Azalea, Cyclamen, Water Hemlock. You can find a list on the DogsTrust website.

Chapter 9
Training At Home

You will need a few tools and some equipment to progress with training and these are outlined below. You will also start by training her some basic cues in the house and in the garden before you start taking her outside for walks. It is always a good idea to cover the basics at home. Here are the main items that you will be using:-

Treats

Treats are the mainstay of dog training at the puppy stage, but you should also introduce other rewards such as toys and praise. In a few cases dogs can prefer toys to treats and I know a Cockapoo who prefers a toy and I would tend to say that this is more unusual..

Some people cut up hot dogs, I made something called liver cake, and one of the simplest things to do is to grab a handful of her kibble and use this as a dog training treat. You will need a selection of 3 or 4 different treats because you will want to adopt a value-reward system.

Value-Reward

A value-reward approach means that you will reward a type of treat based on how difficult the task you are asking her to do is. Kibble, for example, is often not as highly valued as cheese or a piece of hot dog. This means that your puppy will like kibble, but she will like a hot dog more and she will love a small bit of cheese, and she will adore a little bit of liver cake.

In this example, she would get what she loves most when she accomplishes something difficult or that she has never done before. You will then use this knowledge to reward based on difficulty, the more difficult the higher the reward value.

This allows you to reward on value and depending on what you want her to do. You will use this for recall training too, the faster she returns the higher the value of reward. It means that you can use the treat (and later, the reward) that matches her effort.

For example, if she absolutely loves cheese then save this as a special treat when she does something for the first few times. If she has already learned to sit, then offer her kibble when she sits. Try not to move from high value to low value as soon as she learns to sit, gradually move down the value chain to kibble. This process can also increase the connection between you and your puppy and don't forget that you will be praising her all the time.

There are a few reasons that treats might not work. They might not be tasty enough, she might be too stressed or she might get her treats all the time so she doesn't realize what the reward means - this is known as over-reinforcement. It's also possible that your puppy might not be hungry. Try and train her on an empty stomach but not right before she is due to be fed - if a puppy is too hungry then all that her mind will be concentrating on is food and she won't be able to concentrate on her training.

Over reinforcement, which simply means using treats too often, is common. This can be hard to get right but using the value reward system can help. Over-time, rather than getting kibble for example she will get lots of praise and no treat, or her treat might be to do something she loves (play or get the ball) as well as lots of praise.

You are eventually aiming to have the desired behavior with no treats at all and this also helps because you won't always be able to have a treat in your hand.

Harness

Collars and choke collars are no longer thought to be good for dogs. They can be worn in the house but a harness should be used for training - especially leash and recall. Training is all about trust, and restrictive items just won't build the trust you are looking for.

Leash

Avoid flexible leashes. They won't give you the control that you need and they get tangled up in legs including yours or someone else in the park. You will ideally use a long-leash (around 25ft-30ft in length). This is known as a long-line. You will also want a shorter training leash or around 4ft and you can use this as her day-leash or 'normal' leash.

Whistles and Clickers

Almost all leash training will involve using a clicker - I train with and without a clicker. Whistles are great for recall especially for dog breeds that like to explore.

With clicker training, this must always be followed with a reward, for example, click-treat. This is known as the primary and secondary enforcer.

Toys

You are going to use your puppy's toys during recall training. You are aiming to get her to leave a toy and come to you when she is called. You will have a treat so that she sees the value of leaving her toy and coming to you instead.

Basic Training

You can begin basic training over the first few weeks that your puppy is home by teaching her the basic commands that you will use throughout her life.

Always keep the training sessions to between 5 and 10 minutes. If she comes up against something she can't do, then return to something that she can do. You always want her to enjoy the training session so if she gets stuck, take her back a step so that, at the end of the session as well as during it, she is happy and receives her praise and reward - it is important to end the session on a positive note.

I will mention using hand signals during some of the training in the following pages, and you should try to use this type of training as much as you can, rather than only verbal cues. Use both if you don't feel comfortable with only hand signals.

Reinforcement (a part of operant conditioning) and using body language rather than verbal cues is now considered as the foundation for good dog training. Reinforcement is rewarding without a treat i.e. by using praise and offering your puppy something else she loves (a toy or to go and play).

Getting to know her name

Always reward your puppy when she responds to her name. It doesn't matter how or why she responds to her name, it only matters that she does, and you need to reward her for doing so. You will start to do this as soon as she arrives home.

Whenever you say her name and she looks at you, even if it was an accidental look, reward her.

Don't ever be tempted to use her name as punishment because she won't understand and she will be confused by your use of her name and by your annoyance.

Paying Attention

The next stage is to teach her to look at you and you will do this before you start taking your puppy outdoors for walks. I know dogs that, to this day, don't make eye contact with their owner. It is an often overlooked training activity and yet it is a hidden gem in terms of getting your puppy, and later your grown-up dog's, attention and it will make her training much easier.

It will mean that, even if your puppy starts to get engrossed or fixated on something, you can get her attention back to you, and you can change her focus to you, to stop her doing whatever it was that she was doing. I find this particularly useful for leash training.

To do this she needs to want to pay attention to you.

You will already have started training her to look at you during the period you were teaching her her name, but now you want to actively encourage it and to repeat the process in many different locations and environments. You will say her name, she needs to look at you and as soon as she makes eye contact, then you can reward her with click-treat, or with praise and reward, and the reward could be a treat or to play with a toy (Cockapoos love a ball throw, but try to avoid a tennis ball which can rub down her teeth over time, a rubber ball is best).

Training game

A game is the best way to train your Cockapoo to look at you.

To play the game, sit down with your puppy with a handful of treats in your pocket. Make sure that you are sitting so that you are close to her, but that she needs to look up to see your eyes.

Take out a treat and get her attention. Place the treat between your eyes. Your puppy will follow the treat all the way to your head and eyes. As soon as there is eye-contact, even briefly, give her the treat.

In the beginning, the eye contact might be an accident on her part but that's okay. If she gets rewarded for it, she will soon learn. Keep repeating until she always has eye contact with you. If she doesn't look at you at first, then help her find your eyes so that she knows what he is supposed to do.

Once she knows what the game is and is responding in the way that you want, start putting the treat behind your head or neck and try so that she can't see the treat. Again, as soon as there is eye contact - but not before - give her the treat.

The next part of this game is to start using her name. Do exactly the same process but as you place the treat between your eyes, say her name. You will need to do all this quite quickly to link the eye contact with the name call and her reward but she will get there.

She now knows that when you say her name you want her to look at you, and she will want to pay attention to you because there will be a reward coming!

The fundamental cues

You will begin teaching your puppy what you mean by the recall cue. I will use the example of 'come'. The important part is to always use this word and use it only when you want her to come to you. Don't mix it into other cues. This one word means one thing, and one thing only - to come to you.

You will adopt this rule for all her cues. Make sure each one is unique to the action expected and not mixed into other meanings or cues. For example, don't use 'come here' if 'here' is used as another cue.

Start your training in the house then move to enclosed areas with few distractions.

Sit

There are a few ways to teach your puppy to sit, but I have used this one to the best effect.

Sit down beside your puppy holding a treat, then put the treat in front of her nose, slowly lifting it above her head. As she tilts her head up to follow the treat, she is likely to sit as she tries to reach the treat.

You say the word 'sit' just before her bottom touches the ground. Then, as soon as her bottom touches the ground, reward her with the treat. Your puppy is learning the word sit but also starting to recognize your hand signal i.e. the movement of your arm.

Keep doing this, eventually removing the treat from your hand but using your hand as a signal or cue to get her to sit, and saying the word 'sit' as you raise your hand to the sitting position. Always reward her as soon as she sits down.

Don't try to push her bottom to the ground to get her to sit - it rarely works.

Lie Down

For some reason, this is the fastest command to teach when you do it like this, and your puppy will be lying down within one training session.

Simply take out her treat and hold it to her nose, then move it down slowly to the floor (I usually say 'Lie Down' at this point too rather than wait until later in training). Slide the treat on the floor away from her. She will start to move down.

As soon as she is almost down (she won't lie down right away, and her bottom is likely to remain in mid-air), gave her the treat.

Keep doing this and getting her to move further into the lie position (you can keep dragging the treat towards you on the floor as this can often help).

Reward and praise her each time. Eventually, you will only give her the treat when he is fully down. By now, she will be used to your hand moving down and hearing the phrase 'Lie Down.'

Training sit-stay

To teach your dog to stay, first of all, ask her to sit. Then hold up your hand so that your palm is straight in front of her and directed towards her face (but not in any kind of threatening way).

Take a step backward so that you are facing her with your palm facing her and say 'stay'. If she stays for even a few seconds, come back to her and reward her.

Do this a few times and then take a few more steps backward increasing the distance then walk back to her and reward her. Keep repeating moving further away.

Your puppy is learning that not only is he getting rewarded but that you come back to her. Start to move to different positions so that you are to each side and eventually behind her. If she gets up, just move back to her and give her praise then try again.

You will need to repeat this in several different locations not only in one room or only in your own garden. As she starts to get better at this, begin to introduce her to areas with more distractions and start moving behind objects so that she can't see you. Try and do this everywhere you go.

Remember to make sure that you provide the praise/treat when she is sitting and not when she has moved to a standing position. Whenever you puppy sits for you, praise and reward her (with voice or clicker - click-treat) and then start introducing the verbal cue. You can start the verbal cue earlier, for example, say the cue 'sit' right before her bottom touches the ground and she is due to receive his praise/reward.

Every time after that, when your puppy sits try and remember to praise/reward her as she will build this into a behavior default. One that she will enjoy, feels safe with, and knows will bring praise/reward.

The 'come' cue

I know of someone who began basic recall in their hallway, which was ideal for ensuring their puppy was set up for success during the early training because there were limited directional options, and little distraction. This is important. Remember that you want to ensure that your puppy always succeeds and this might mean you need to adapt things to make sure that he can succeed through each step of his training.

Once you have decided on your location, show your puppy her favorite treat or toy, and as she comes towards you to get her toy or treat (don't ask her to come to you, let her do it by herself), praise her and reward her as he reaches you. Do this a few times.

Once again, add some distraction. One fun way to do this is to have other family members or friends in a room with you. As you walk towards them and she starts to get interested in this interesting and fun distraction, quickly run away and call her so that she chases you.

Encourage her to catch up and when she does, she will of course get his treat and probably a big cuddle as an extra reward.

Like many of the training games you can play with her, mix them up so that she doesn't always know what to expect. It will keep her even more interested in what you are about to get up to next.

After a few times start to add in her cue so that she gets used to it. As she starts coming towards you to get her toy (and ideally looks at you), add in the cue you have chosen. In my example, 'Come'. Once she is doing this you can add in a sit.

Combine sit, stay and come

Finally, combine the 'come' cue with the 'sit and stay' cue.

This was the main recall training I started with Millie indoors when she was around 14 weeks old and it was very effective.

Ask your puppy to sit, and then ask her to stay - I also held my hand up as a 'stay' visual cue..

Walk backwards a few steps while facing your puppy - I kept holding my hand up as I was walking away.

The difference now is that you want her to come to you following the sit-stay. If she stays for just a few seconds, ask her to come and give her a treat and be delighted with her.

Keep repeating this and do it at the start of every training session. As she starts to get good at this, start to move further and further away and eventually try walking away with your back to her.

Like all of her training, build up the distance and the distractions to this game - but if you go too far and she starts to come towards you too soon, just go back a few steps to the point at which it was working and then keep trying to build the distance.

The next stage is to go outside but not for a 'proper' walk just yet. You can go for a walk on-leash but not off-leash.

Summary and the 10 steps for basic recall

1. Decide on your location (hallway, kitchen, etc) - and later, vary the location
2. Show your puppy her favorite toy or a treat but don't call her, let her come to you
3. When she gets to you give her the treat along with praise
4. Repeat
5. Start adding your recall cue ('come', visual cue or whistle) as she starts coming towards you
6. Reward her when she gets to you
7. Repeat steps 5 and 6
8. When she comes to you give her the treat then ask her to sit and give her another treat
9. Repeat this until she knows what to do
10. Ask her to sit and stay, walk away from her and then use her cue to come to you
11. When she gets to you give her the treat along with praise
12. Repeat the recall and sit and stay in other locations and start to add in distractions

Leash training

You can start putting her lead on in the house so that she gets used to it. As soon as her leash is clipped on, give her a treat. Have another treat in your hand and use this to get her to walk beside you.

To do this, hold the treat just in front of her nose, loosely cupped in your hand, so that your palm is facing her nose with your arm hanging down beside you.

She will move towards your hand as you start taking a few steps forward which makes her move and walk along beside you. Build this up slowly and for no more than 5 minutes at a time at the start.

Eventually, walk a few paces, then turn in the opposite direction getting her to follow you.

Repeat this process of walking a few steps and turning.

Chapter 10
Recall Training

In this chapter we will outline the main training you will start doing with your puppy as you prepare, and then, start taking her out for walks.

Cues

Dogs train better when they are making their own choices. You want her to want to make the choice to come to you, when you ask her. This means that you must never be angry when she comes back to you, no matter how long it has taken.

You are aiming to have your dog return to you on cue no matter how many other exciting things are going on around her. This means that your puppy needs to want to return to you on cue, not only when there are no other dogs around, but also when there are dogs to play with.

You can only achieve this if you are more interesting than whatever else she is doing, and if she is listening, and paying attention to you.

In summary, you want her to stop what she is doing; you want her to look at you, and you want her to come to you on cue.

Introducing the recall cue

Most people use the word 'come' or 'here' as their vocal cue for their recall. Some might use a whistle. I mix a verbal and visual cue. Once you have decided on the word you want to use, then you must keep it. Consistency is vital for your dog to understand what you mean.

You will start using this early. When you want her to come for her dinner you will use it, and when you are going to give her a big cuddle or play with her, you will use it.

The outcome of her action when she hears the word and responds correctly means she feels great because she gets something she loves and she gets lots of praise from you. In dog training language, she is building a positive association with the word.

Try to build in hand signals too - I tend to open my arms as a visual cue to come.

Like most training sessions, keep the training to around 10 minutes and watch out for any signs that she is getting stressed (quick head movements, grabbing the treat/food, ears flat) and try not to get her over-excited.

If your puppy is a part of a household then get all members involved in the training too. Don't forget to ask her to do something you know she can do at the end of the training so that it ends in success. You want her to enjoy her training.

You will have already introduced her to training at home including the basic 'sit', 'stay, and 'come' cues. You will now begin leash and recall training in preparation for her daily walks and exercise in the park.

You won't let her off leash outside in an unenclosed area until you are happy that she will return to you.

To do this you need to introduce her to different locations and train her in these locations - different rooms in the house, different areas of the garden or different areas of an enclosed area. You will then introduce lots of distractions as the training develops - a toy, another person, another dog that you know (and that you know is vaccinated) etc and you will keep doing the training exercises with all these distractions present.

You are aiming to get her to always pay attention to you and to always return to you despite any exciting activity or scents that she might be interested in - and if she can get used to this in a safe garden then she will be familiar with what to do once she gets to the park.

When it comes to recall, you should wait until her recall is up to about 70%-80% before you start adding the distraction element of her recall training.

Sit Stay Release

Sit Stay is one of the most important cues your dog will learn and the ones you will use most often.

You will want to use both verbal and visual cues. Your visual cue for 'stay' will be holding up your hand, but without raising your arm above your head - just hold it in front of you and direct your palm to your puppy's face. This is his visual cue for stay.

The verbal cue would be 'Stay'. Visual cues are also a good way of helping your dog focus on you.

Normally the first part is to ask your puppy to 'sit' then this is followed by 'stay' (or 'wait').

By this stage (by the time you are going for outside walks) you will have trained your puppy to 'sit' and will have practiced some 'stay' in the home or garden. We have covered this earlier.

You will now start to use the sit cue for a variety of reasons. In the car, when you go to the door, when you are at a crosswalk, and so on. This means you need to train her to sit but you also need to let her know when it's okay to move forward.

To do this, first of all, have her on the leash. Get her to sit (and reward) then decide on your cue for 'let's go' this can be 'let's go' or 'ok go' or whatever you choose. Say your cue and move a few steps and praise her, ask her to sit and reward.

Begin with short distances (a few steps) to get her used to the 'ok go' cue. Repeat the process of 'sit', reward 'ok go' reward, walk a few steps then repeat. This is known as the release cue.

This can mean that the release cue is seen as a reward too because when she comes back she then gets to go and have fun again. It also means that she will learn that coming back doesn't mean the end of the play.

Finally, some trainers consider recall to include holding your puppy's collar when she returns as full recall and they use it before the release cue. The puppy comes back, she sits and the collar is taken then the reward is given. This is followed by the release cue.

Some are happy with only the sit. This really is up to you but I prefer the collar hold as it gives you more control should you ever need it.

Training Outside

Training for recall outside of the house is vital. It is here that she is going to find the most distractions. You must make sure that the area you choose is fully enclosed. Just like the early days of house training, you will start with very few distractions.

This is when you are going to work with the clicker and training leads and when you will start working out the value that she attaches to each of her different treats if you haven't already done so.

A great tip is to train your puppy before she has eaten - this means the treat you are offering will be of higher value to her and she will be more interested in them! And don't train her for too long. Pay attention if she looks like she is getting bored and stop the training and start again the next day.

To get started, put your puppy in her harness and on her training leash. Just like the early indoor training, you can start with rewarding an action with no other cues, to get her used to the long-line and outdoor training. She will know what to do quickly, because she has already been trained indoors.

The difference now is that you are going to place something she might want to eat or might want to get (a toy), a short distance away from her, and within the length of the leash, or just a bit further away. You are now introducing something she wants to get to, that is away from you.

As she goes towards the object or the treat (but not too tasty), tighten her leash and say her name then the cue e.g., Millie 'come'. As soon as she turns and comes (even if it's only a step or two) reward and praise her.

If you are using a clicker, you will click as soon as she turns (there is more on clicker training later). Aim to have an even tastier treat for her than the one she was going towards. You want to increase the value of the treats the more you want her to do something, so that she prefers to choose that treat.

By having the leash on her, you can also gently encourage her to come towards you to get her reward if you need to. The leash helps you have a bit of control over this recall in the early stages as she continues to establish the cue 'come' outside of the house, and where she will want to explore.

You will also play on the training leash and long line. Give her a few treats then run forward or backward a few steps and say 'Millie, Come!' in a playful voice while holding a treat out at the height of her nose (so that all of her feet are on the ground) and as she reaches you give her the treat.

You can extend this game to add the sit. As she reaches you to get her treat, move the treat up in front of her nose, so that she is forced back into the sit position to get her treat. In this way the come and sit are the same cue which means when you ask her to come, she will come to you and sit without being asked to sit.

You can, and should start practicing this as soon as you can. Puppies learn most up to the age of 18 weeks.

The next step for recall training is to have her move further away from you, and for her to return when she hears her cue. Good recall means she does this all the time. If she is not, then he is not ready, and you won't want to risk letting her off-leash. You will have already trained her to come and you are now continuing to establish this outside of the home.

To understand what you are asking your puppy to do, think about it like this. She is exploring and having fun, she is finding interesting and exciting things to sniff and play with. When you call her, you want her to prefer to come to you rather than to do whatever she is doing. If you can achieve this, then there is no reason for her not to return to you when called.

To do this you will want to start including training games, you will have worked out what her favorite treats are, and which ones top the list. Cheese, hotdog, carrot, kibble - my two dogs love cheese and I used to make liver cake which they absolutely loved. It was probably the single reason Millie's recall and leash training went so well.

Using the long-line

You don't need to use the long-line but it can be really helpful and, if you can, I would recommend it. To describe how this is done I picked a hand but you will end up doing something that works for you.

Practice this in a garden if you can, and, in the beginning, have no other distractions. You want to get used to working with the long line and you also want to test that your training is working.

Hold the end of the line in your right hand so that you have it tightly held. Wrap the length of the line into loops so that you can slowly release the line over the front of your body, feeding it through your left hand, making sure it can be easily released.

In your left hand, you are holding the part of the line that is acting as your dog leash, and it is attached to her harness, and your hand is operating as a feeder, controlling the delivery of the line.

This means you can slowly release the line through your left hand, to allow your puppy to move away from you, or clamp it closed (gently) to stop further release of the line.

You will have your right hand holding the end of the long line as well as the loops of the spare line. Once you are comfortable you can start the training.

Slowly move in a circle on the same spot so that she is running around you, loosening the line so that she can move away from you, and then call her back to you. Just get her used to the leash and watching you, and knowing that she gets a reward when she comes back.

You can then add another game (and later you can play this off-leash too), by throwing a treat away from you, and letting your puppy go towards the treat.

Once she has eaten her treat, call her name to get her attention, wait until she looks at you (click), 'come' (cue), and when she comes to you (praise/reward). Then throw another treat in a different direction so that she is constantly running away and towards you in a fun game.

When you need to tighten or 'pull' the line to encourage her to come back on her cue, move or lean forward rather than move against her, and gently make the line shorter. This allows you to be in control of your puppy whilst letting her return without feeling 'pulled'.

The final part is to wait until she is preoccupied with something and is not looking at you. Get her attention and ask her to come. If she comes then praise and reward. If she doesn't come, just walk to her and show her all the treats you have, and then walk away from her.

She is likely to follow you to try and get a treat. Just ignore her. As soon as she isn't right beside you, ask her to come to you. When she does, give her lots of praise and a favorite treat. It won't take long for her to realize that coming is much better than not coming.

The next step is to repeat the indoor sit stay come training in the outdoor environment. Just as you did indoors get your puppy to sit-stay and then move away from her while still facing her and then ask her to 'come'. e.g., 'Millie, come'. Slowly build the distance all the while using the long line.

The next two steps are new, and before you can try off-leash outdoor you want to introduce the 'let's go' or 'let's play' cue which combines the sit-stay.

Ask her to sit-stay beside you, then use your release cue, 'let's go', and start walking. As he moves away and then moves ahead of you, call her back to you (click on a turn of the head towards you), as he starts coming towards you might want to encourage her (I held my arms open), reward her when he gets to you, then ask her to sit (reward).

The last step is to practice off-leash - again, you will do this in a space that is enclosed and where he will be safe. Simply let her wander away from you and then call her to you using your cue. Be exciting and have a treat ready for her. Try and keep his attention on you as he comes to you - make a noise or hold your arms open - you want her to be focused on you.

Don't keep repeating the cue or start raising your voice if he doesn't come. This will confuse her, and he won't be able to understand what his cue word is, eventually tuning it out which means he just won't hear it.

If you raise your voice, he won't think that coming to you is going to be lots of fun. Eventually, it could have the opposite effect, and he won't want to come at all.

The best way to train your puppy is using random and variable reinforcement. All this means is that over time change how often he gets a treat for the same behavior, so that he is hoping for it each time (don't wait too long to reward as you start to reduce the level of treats) and change the value of the treat (for a really good response).

If you want to, you can measure the average response time for recall (either daily or per 12 returns, etc.) so that when he comes back faster, he gets a super tasty treat. This is the most effective way to train your puppy to become addicted to coming back to you.

One last trick - if your puppy has taken a while to return on cue then, when he arrives, show her the treat and put it back in your pocket. As he moves away ask her to 'come' and, when he gets to you, give her his treat. This will help her learn that acting right away gets the reward.

Using a Clicker

Clicker training is useful when you want to mark the correct behavior of your puppy at the exact moment that she starts to respond. If you are doing click-reward then it must always be followed by a reward, but the reward and the timing of the reward varies.

In the beginning, all you need to do is get your puppy used to the click-reward (at the start you will use a treat). Keep repeating click-treat. She doesn't have to do anything at this stage as you are just getting her used to the clicker marker which means a reward is coming.

Slowly reduce the time between the click and the treat and vary the gaps - she will still expect the treat and he will know that it is coming, but that it might not happen right away.

Once she gets good at this, you will be able to click without the treat, and vary the reinforcement by using hers favorite toy or a quick game that she likes.

For example, when you call her name and she begins to start coming towards you, you can click so that she knows a reward is coming. It helps to keep her motivated to come all the way back to you in the expectation of a good time when she gets there.

Below is how clicker training fits in to the training so far as well as how it its in to recall. If you are trining without a clicker just ignore the click-marker.

Recall Summary and where the Clicker fits in

The general process for recall training is as follows:

1. Call your dog (use your 'come' cue)
2. When she comes ask her to "Sit" (cue). Take her collar and praise her and reward
3. Release her "Ok Go" (cue)

If you are using a clicker as a marker then the complete process would look like this:

Get your puppy to come to you

Start by throwing a treat away from you then throw a treat at your feet. Reward every time your puppy comes back to you for any reason. You can add the click with your clicker to mark as soon as she turns towards you.

Add a cue

As your puppy turns towards you, again, this is for any reason, add your recall cue and your click (if you are using a clicker to mark or capture the behavior). The recall cue can be 'come', 'here' or a whistle - either your own whistle or use a plastic one.

As you are walking on the leash vary the length. Every time she looks towards you, click and then add the recall cue (and don't forget the reward). Practice at different locations and over different distances before you move to the next step.

You will now cue her to look and come to you. With your puppy walking in front of you say (or whistle) your cue, as she turns towards you add the click marker. Practice by varying the distance and the speed the dog is moving away. When she returns to you reward.

If you want to add a sit then this is when you will add it to your training. When she arrives back to you use your sit cue to get her to sit. As soon as she sits add a click and then the reward.

Add a collar hold

You can train this separately or you can add it into the recall process here. When she has arrived back and sits, lean in and take hold of her collar - as you do this use your clicker to mark then reward.

Once she is good and is succeeding with these steps you can start adding in distractions.

Distractions

You will start with low-level distractions and build them up to higher-value distractions.

Distractions might be kibble, bread, eggs, cheese, meat, and toys (again in order of least to most favorite).

As she moves towards the distraction e.g., the bread, start your recall cue, and the reward process above (if you are using a clicker just add the click marker). If she fails then reduce the value of the distraction until she is succeeding.

In terms of what distractions might be, then this can be a dog she knows, a dog she doesn't know (high-value distraction), someone she knows, a group of people, a jogger, a bicycle an old scent, and the high-value new scent (a squirrel that you have noticed running up a tree).

Try and remember to complete a sequence. Try to always have your dog notice you (click), come to you (encouragement), arrive (treat), sit (treat), collar hold (treat), 'go play' (reward). This is much more rewarding than 'come', treat, end of the game.

By continuing to reward after she comes back to you, by rewarding the sit, collar hold and then releasing with a 'go play' cue, she will have the expectation of more exciting things to come than if the rewards ended with the return cue only.

She also knows that she can return to playing if she comes back to you and also receives all of her rewards. Don't forget that the 'go play' cue is a reward in itself.

This will become even more useful once you start going outdoors to parks and other walks where there are even more exciting distractions and ones that you are not in control of.

Proofing

Proofing is when you want to 'prove' that the training has worked and you will need to do this before you let your puppy off-leash.

To do this, you will create distractions and then aim to get her to come to you on cue.

Try and arrange a play-date with at least one other dog and then while she is playing with it (and still on the long-line) call her to you. Make sure you have a very tasty treat and be full of praise when she comes to you.

Once she comes to you and receives her reward she is then released to the cue, such as 'let's go', to play again. As already mentioned, this particular activity is also useful to teach her that coming to you doesn't mean the end of the playtime.

The last step is to practice off-leash - again, you will do this in a space that is enclosed and where she will be safe. Simply let her wander away from you and then call her to you using your cue. Be exciting and have a treat ready for her.

Don't keep repeating the cue if she doesn't come and don't raise your voice to a shout (or scream). This will confuse her and she won't be able to understand what her cue word is. If you raise your voice, she won't think that coming to you is going to be lots of fun and it can have the opposite effect, and she won't want to come at all.

If she isn't coming to you as you go through all the training then go back to the long line until you are sure she understands what you are asking her to do.

Emergency stop

Training for an emergency stop save your dog's life. It is also quite easy to train especially once you have been working on recall training.

First of all, you will want to use a specific cue. This can be any word but, again, it can only have one meaning. The most common word that is used is 'Stop'.

To begin with, have your puppy sitting in front of you and have a treat in your hand. If your puppy is not food orientated try using one of her toys.

Take a step back, put your arm in the air as if you are trying to stop the traffic or saying hello to someone who is a distance away. This is important as it is more likely that your emergency stop signal will be visual and not sound-based because your dog is more likely to be a distance away from you.

Raise your arm with the treat in your hand, say the word 'Stop', and then throw the treat over your dog's head towards his rear so that the treat falls behind her or just beside her. You want to make sure that your dog needs to turn around to get the treat.

As she starts to return to you, repeat by putting your arm in the air, saying 'Stop' and throwing another treat over his head. This will force her to stop to turn around to get the treat.

You will notice that she starts to pay attention to you and your hand, which is what you want her to do.

Once she is paying attention, stopping and turning to get the treat as you raise your arm, you can think about increasing the distance of your throw. If there are any problems with the next step return to this previous stage.

Keep throwing the treat a bit further away so that there is a bigger distance between you both, so that when you say 'Stop', put your arm in the air, and throw the treat over her head, she is not close to you. This is how you can build up the long-distance emergency stop.

Try to make sure the treat doesn't land in front of her because you want her to turn around to get the treat. You want her to do this because it stops her forward movement. Keep building up the distance and repeating the exercise.

You want to reach the point where, with your arm in the air, you say Stop, she looks towards you and stops. If she starts to come towards you, go back to the first step and reinforce the Stop when she is right in front of you.

If your dog is a fast learner it may take a few days but this can take a few weeks so just be patient.

The very last step is when you don't throw the treat at the end but, instead, you walk towards her to give her the reward. This is because, if you are in a park and she is far away, you won't be able to throw a treat behind her but you want her to know that a reward is coming.

What not to do

If your dog does not return to you when you call her simply go and retrieve her and put her on her leash. Don't be angry with her, simply put her on the leash, and move her away from whatever it is that is distracting her. This, in itself, lets her know that coming back is a much better option.

Don't keep calling the same cue over and over again. For example, if she does not come when you call and you keep repeating the cue louder and louder the cue itself will lose its value and your puppy will simply tune it out as noise. If your cue isn't working then choose a new one and train your puppy to know what it is.

Don't have only one person training her if dhe lives with other family members. If your puppy is a family dog then everyone needs to be involved in the training, and everyone needs to use the same cues. Ideally, everyone should be involved in the daily training, even for just a few minutes.

Never punish your puppy when she fails. This is particularly important with recall (and with separation anxiety). If you get angry with them, or punish them, when they finally return to you after not coming back right away, all they will learn is that coming back to you is not a good experience and that it has negative consequences. It is not fun. All this will do is make his recall worse, not better.

Don't use the "come" cue if your dog if fully focused on something else and is unlikely to 'hear' you. In this case, use her name to get her attention and to check that she can hear you (does she react by turning slightly towards you or twitch her ear). If she does, then use her "come" cue. If she is far away you can use a whistle or whistle yourself, and if she can see you use your hand signal.

Only use your "come" cue if you think it is likely to succeed. If you call and she does not come, walk to her. Don't give her into trouble or reward her. If she does not 'come' you know she is not fully trained so re-start the training to the point she was succeeding, and build it up again from there.

Finally, do no use the recall cue for things they might not like doing. For example, don't associate it with a bath, or getting groomed, or having a tick removed of they don;t like these things.

Chapter 11
Park Life

Once you are ready to go to the park you are going to encounter even more distractions and you will want to begin with using high value (or higher value) treats than you have been using indoors and in the enclosed area.

It is going to be harder for her to return, and therefore you want the reward to be extra special. You will also vary these treats so she doesn't know what to expect but she knows a really tasty treat is coming.

You might also want to vary the timing of the treat so she knows it's coming and it will be tasty but it might be in 1, 2, or 5 seconds (you will want to start varying the immediacy of the reward when you are doing the outdoor enclosed training).

Try not to only call your dog to you at the end of her walk. If you do it throughout the walk and reward her each time she comes back, she won't associate recall with the end of playtime.

At the end of the walk, make coming back fun and rewarding rather than something she doesn't like. I tend to play more at the end of the walk as I return to the entry gate of the park.

During the walk, you can vary her treat reward depending on how well she comes back to you when you give her the recall cue. If you call, and she continues to do what she is doing for a minute or two and then comes back, don't reward her right away. Let her smell her treat and then let her start to move away from you. Call her again quickly (you want her to succeed) and if she immediately turns around and comes back then reward and praise her.

In the early stages, try rewarding her with one of her less favorite treats rather than no reward at all for taking her time to come back. You want to ensure that she doesn't think he is being punished (by not getting her treat) for coming back, even if she took her time about it.

If you have already established a connection with your puppy and he finds you interesting, this will be much easier.

You can take your puppy to the park on a long line but never let her off-leash until you are confident of her recall - even if you have proofed, the first time you take her you will want to start slowly. You can let go of the long line and if she runs too far you can stand on the end of it. It is much easier to do this than try and grab a shorter lead.

As you start to venture out on walks, your puppy won't be the only one meeting other similar animals to talk and play with.

It's important to pay attention to your puppy and to keep playing with her, and being fun, during a walk too. Standing around and talking to other dog walkers and ignoring her will mean, although she might be well exercised through all her running around, she is learning that you are not the most exciting thing in her life and her attention to you (and your recall cue) may not be 'heard'. She will simply tune it out as her attention will be elsewhere.

Other dogs and their communication signals

The first thing that is going to happen when you can take your puppy out for real walks after her required vaccinations, is that she is going to meet other dogs that you both don't know.

Your puppy is going to be playful and excited to meet other dogs, but these dogs may not be so eager to have an excited puppy trying to play with them.

Older dogs (those over 2 years old) are not likely to want to play - in fact - dogs over 2 years old will tend to only play with dogs they know. Many will stop playing with other dogs altogether. Both Millie and Barney don't play with other dogs anymore, they run along together or play with their balls or sticks.

You will also need to pay attention to how the dogs you meet are reacting. Dogs will tell you far in advance if they are getting annoyed, are uncomfortable or feel threatened. I don't know how many times I have seen the owner of a dog watch as his dog tries to get another dog to play, and the dog being approached tries, again and again, to say 'no' until eventually, it runs out of options and snaps or even tries to bite to the dog who is pestering it.

These are the general stages to watch out for, and this will be the case both for your dog, and for the dogs that you meet. Try to pay attention to what dogs are telling each other and telling us.

If a dog is displaying this behavior, then these are signs that he is feeling threatened, and is not happy with the attention of another dog, when it is close to her: -

Stage 1: Yawning, looking away, licking lips, moving away

Stage 2: Panting, hackles up, and whale eyes (when a dog shows the whites of his eyes). This is a clear warning signal. If this still doesn't work then the next part will be a lip curl or snarl

Stage 3: Lip curl or snarl or growl and possibly a snap. Then finally we will reach the stage we don't want to be

Stage 4: A lunge towards the other dog (or the source of the 'threat') with barking as your dog tries to make the threat go away and then this may be followed by a bite.

How dogs greet each other

You need to be aware of other dogs and understand what they are saying.

A dog running at another dog is not going to go down well. I am still surprised how often I see dog owners letting their dogs do this. Both Millie and Barney are friendly dogs but they hate it. If you see a dog running towards your puppy or dog, then there are a few things you can do.

As soon as I see this happening, and depending on how far away the other dog is, and how fast they are running, I will throw a ball or a stick to distract Millie and Barney. This can sometimes encourage the other dog as well, and if I notice this, I just ignore the other dog and turn away with Millie and Barney in the opposite direction. If Barney is playing further away from me, and he feels threatened by another dog, he comes back to me to be safe. If a dog runs towards him, he comes as close as he can.

Millie tends to feel less threatened and seems to find it easier to deal with other dogs without resorting to aggression or fear. She must communicate well! She does this by a lip curl, then a growl, sometimes she adds in a whale eye, then an air snap but all of this is extremely unusual and she needs a lot of provocation. Like most dogs, she will always tries avoidance if she can.

Others signs to watch out for include tails, are the tails up, and are the hackles up? Neither necessarily mean that the dog is aggressive but it indicates high adrenaline. If you notice this, distract your puppy or dog away from the other dog.

Two dogs that meet each other head-on and stare into each other's faces are not being friendly, but a dog that approaches from the side is being polite and asking for the intrusion into your dog's space.

A face greeting followed by a bottom sniff tends to be friendly. Bottom sniffing, generally, is fine and nothing to worry about.

If another dog puts his head across another dogs' shoulders this can be a sign of aggression and it can often be followed by mounting.

Just remember to always ask the other dog owner if it is ok for your puppy or dog to play with their dog. Do this especially if their dog is on a leash. Don't forget a dog that is on a leash might feel threatened by another dog, who is not on a leash, and who then tries to play with her. The dog on the leash will feel constrained, and this can lead to anxiety and a reaction to defend herself.

All of this is very important as your puppy begins her first walks. The experiences she has with other dogs at this stage are vital to how she views other dogs in the future, and if her experience is negative then she can easily build a negative association with other dogs - and be aggressive herself because she might see them as a threat.

One of the ways that you can help keep your puppy from getting over-excited around other dogs is to be more exciting yourself! Of course, you can also teach her sit-stay. Every time she sees another dog you will want to get her to sit and stay (and reward and praise her at each stage as she learns this). You can use a clicker if you wish, and every time she learns a little bit more, click and reward.

As you first start to take your puppy out, she is likely to want to run up to other dogs herself. This is very different as it will be clear to most dogs that she is not being aggressive but curious and playful.

However, and as noted earlier, dogs older than 2 years old don't tend to like being harassed by a puppy so just make sure you don't create a situation that then leads your puppy to start fearing other dogs. Millie, who is now 11 years old and has been a mum herself, will persevere with a puppy for a few minutes but she will then let it know to leave her alone. Barney (now 6 years old) will try to completely ignore a puppy for as long as he can.

However, puppies learn by meeting other dogs and learning not to bother them, so try and teach them the basics with a dog you know.

How to interact with humans

You will already know some of these but a couple of points are worth re-stating. Don't let a stranger pat your puppy or dog on the head. They can bring their hand slowly towards them from the side so he can sniff the hand.

If your puppy starts to back away this is a sign of fear, and an early communication, so try to notice it and don't ignore it.

If your puppy starts to yawn, or lick his lips, then this is the next level of communication, and he is really trying to tell you and the other person that he is uncomfortable.

The final warning will be a bark. She will only get to this stage if nothing else has worked.

The best way to try and teach her that someone is not to be feared is to reward your puppy when he sees them to create a positive association. You can also try showing your puppy that there is nothing to fear by touching, perhaps shaking a hand, and quietly talking, and while you are doing this, reward with a high-value treat.

Games

You will use games for lots of reasons. One of the things you want to get your puppy to do is to watch you, and know where you are. You always want to be moving around so that he knows he needs to keep an eye on you all the time.

Hide and go seek is also a great game to play. I love it more than the dogs and you probably will too. This is a fun game that teaches them to pay attention to you. I still play hide and seek with them just to remind them to watch me and know where I am. All you do is hide behind a tree or a wall or any object. Let her run over to you and then come out, praise her and give her his treat. It's really simple but they love it.

A good way to play a game that reinforces paying attention to you (and can help remove any anxiety of other dogs that might be close-by) is to have them walk slightly in front of you and then throw a really nice (and smelly) treat near you both for no apparent reason. This helps your puppy know that you might do something fun when she isn't expecting it.

A game I have found particularly good with my spaniels is ball play. They play with their ball all the time and always need to come back to have me throw it for them. It means when I am out with them, they rarely leave me.

Millie moves between balls, sticks and she loves pine cones (in the winter she loves to find a lost glove). They might surprise you with the things they love to retrieve (I call it 'fetch' and use this word as a cue). Frisbees are also popular and we had a retriever who loved a Frisbee.

Another great game is chase. As the name suggests, as your puppy is coming towards you give them lots of praise and get them to chase you. Most dogs love this game but some just don't have any interest in it, so this will depend on your own puppy. But changing up the reward, and keeping things exciting and different for your puppy is really important or they might get bored with you.

Never play chase the other way around. Never chase your puppy or dog as a game. Chasing teaches her the opposite of what you want for recall (and being able to take hold of her, especially if you need to do it quickly). It will be very confusing for her when she doesn't get rewarded when she runs away from you and it can cause all sorts of problems.

Finally, and one last example of a fun game is piggy in the middle. This is a great game for recall and everyone can join in. As the name suggests, someone calls your puppy's name and gives them a treat or a toy, then someone else calls his name and he runs to them and gets a treat or the toy, and so on. This is actually great fun and a great way to get comfortable when you go to the park for the first time.

Your puppy will let you know what games and toys he likes best.

Chapter 12
General Training Tips

Introducing her to the sitter

Cockapoos, especially if they are from single parent homes, may not like going to a dog sitter or dog walker.

If you are going to use a dog sitter or dog walker then, in the beginning, don't take her to the sitter. It is much better if the sitter comes to your house to pick her up. If you take her to the sitter, you have to 'leave'. If the sitter comes to pick her up then you are 'staying'. Do this until your dog is happy and comfortable with the sitter or walker.

Introducing her to a new home with dogs

If you are going to visit someone who has dogs then you want to introduce her to the other dogs in a neutral environment. It is better to take them all for a walk before you go into the house so that they can get to know each other first.

Activities to avoid until adulthood

Agility training and obstacle courses, and having too many long walks or runs when they are young is not good for your puppy because her joints are not fully mature. Doing too much, too early can cause problems in alter life especially if there is any risk of hip dysplasia. Wait until they have reached adulthood before you take them running with you or you take them to agility classes. Fetch games and swimming are much better for them when they are younger (but not it they like jumping for the ball every time they play fetch).

Excessive Barking

Your Cockapoo can bark for a few reasons:

Guarding: At certain times, barking for guarding is the correct behaviour but your Cockapoo can become overly attached to you and bark at friends and family when they are around you.

Offensive/Defensive: This can happen in the park or if a new dog is introduced to your Cockapoo. This is most likely because your Cockapoo is nervous or lacks confidence. They might see these encounters as a threat to their safety and so they bark to scare it away (defensive) or warn of an attack (offensive).

Boredom/Attention Seeking: As we know, Cockapoos are very intelligent and this means that they can get bored easily and start seeking your attention if you are not focused on them. This can lead to barking and nipping (or chewing). This problem can be reinforced because when they behave like this, they get more attention.

Excited: Cockapoos (and Cockers Spaniels) can bark when they are excited.

The first step is to identify which reason is causing this behaviour - and it could also be separation anxiety which we discuss in the following chapter.

If the reason is either separation anxiety or boredom and attention seeking then you will focus on the cause. In terms of boredom and attention then the easiest way to deal with this is to give her games to play that can keep her occupied. You want games that test her mind such as getting food out of a Kong or a ball out of a box.

For guarding and offensive/defensive barking, then you want to use positive training to tackle the problem. Whatever you do, don't shout at her to stay quiet because this will make her believe that the 'threat' is even greater.

Try to introduce a place for her in the home - a place where she can go to - this can be her basket or her cage. If she starts to bark when someone new is in the home (or when the doorbell rings), you will ignore her until she stops, then you will ask her to go to her 'basket'. You want to get her attention (deflection) and then will give her a reward. You then want to ask her to go to her basket and when she does you need to make a fuss of her and give her a treat. You are aiming to train her to go to her 'safe place' and it may take a few weeks. If she is reacting to visitors in your home, then you might also have the person who is visiting give her a treat.

If she is reacting to other dogs, then deflection is the best way to re-direct her energy. Get her attention by asking her to do something - you are only trying to take her attention away from the other dog. Give her the ball, or ask her to sit and reward her.

Don't reward her for simply stopping barking. You want her to do something that you ask of her, so that she doesn't confuse the reward with the barking you are trying to stop!.

If all of this fails, then believe it or not, teaching her to bark on cue might help. This is because you will ask her to bark and then ask her to 'be quiet'. I have used the cue 'speak' then a reward, then 'quiet' then a reward. It can be a remarkably fast way to insert yourself into her barking and getting her to know that you want it to stop.

Chapter 13
Separation Anxiety

Cockapoos are prone to suffer from separation anxiety and, because of this, it should form a part of all Cockapoo puppy training.

But Cockapoos are not alone, separation anxiety affects at least 1 in 7 dogs in the United States with some studies reporting it might be as high as 1 in 5.

The very best thing you can do, if you have a new puppy or a newly adopted dog, is to train your pup as soon as you can.

Separation training is not generally top of the training list for new puppy parents - we all know that we need to teach sit, stay, leash and potty training - but we need to add separation training to that list. It is one of the most important training exercises that can ensure that both you and your dog can have a happy life and one that teaches her that it is okay to be home alone.

Separation Anxiety can be a form of separation distress or isolation distress - a milder form of separation anxiety. I use the terms separation anxiety as a general term but it will depend on the depth of the issue for your dog.

It happens when a dog reacts to separation (usually when their 'family' leaves the home) and this results in your dog getting stressed. This stress is released in a variety of ways, from whining and barking, to chewing and destruction, with a few poops in between.

This chapter is not intended for those dogs with serious anxiety problems, but rather as a guide, to help with some of the basic steps to ease your dog's anxiety with separation - and to also explain why they feel the way they do.

Dogs are used to living with others. They are pack animals, and in nature, are never alone. As man's best friend this means their pack includes us and everyone else we may live within our homes. In its simplest form, being 'separate' is not a natural experience for a dog.

Humans can, and do, live more separately. We are used to it because we need to do things like go to work, we might need to go to school or we just need to go shopping. We are therefore asking our dogs to behave unnaturally. This means that we need to teach them how to live in our world where some form of separation is a necessity.

Try to remember that for us our dogs, no matter how much we love them, are our pets. But, to them, we are a part of their pack. They see us as their family. They make no distinction between being human or not. And so it is natural for them to be with us and to follow us around - just like they would do with their pack.

There are a few theories on why dogs react the way that they do but the most important thing to know is that if they are suffering from any degree of separation anxiety then, for one reason or another, they are getting stressed when you leave and they are being left alone. All we need to do is to help teach them that being alone without you is not to be feared.

Dogs are not the same

Separation or canine separation anxiety can affect all dogs, although research suggests that dogs are more likely to develop separation behavior problems if they are male, come from a shelter, or are separated from the litter before they are 60 days old.

Interestingly, dogs born at home were more likely to suffer anxiety than those born with a breeder. This might explain why Barney, who was born at home, is more anxious than his mother, Millie.

Separation anxiety can, and does, occur for other reasons. It also happens to older dogs as well as with puppies.

Dogs that tend to have higher levels of alertness, which are more common in some types of breeds than others, are also thought to increase the chance of that dog experiencing separation anxiety. The Cockapoo is in prime territory here.

In research, mixed breed dogs like Cockapoos were more likely to destroy, urinate or defecate when left alone, whereas, for example, Wheaten Terriers were likely to vocalize, salivate or pant. Where separation anxiety existed, almost all of the dogs also had a fear of noise. Miniature Schnauzers and Staffordshire Bull Terriers were the least affected by noise.

However, not all Cockapoos will develop separation anxiety, it just means that they are more susceptible to it.

Signs Of Separation Anxiety

Separation anxiety is not a failure on the owner's part, and there can be many reasons that a dog reacts like this.

There may have been a change in ownership either from another home or from a shelter, there may have been a house move or a change in the routine of the family, it might be due to divorce or the loss of a family member (usually another dog but it could be a cat or even a family member moving away to school).

For puppy's, it might simply be the first time they have been left alone having been used to being around people all the time.

Dogs may also have had a bad experience - firecrackers, a delivery person, or the noise from trash pick-up. Dogs don't like sudden and unexpected noises.

Like anyone, dogs can get more nervous if they are alone. But remember, dogs are not used to dealing with threats alone, they are used to packs who are there for safety as well as nurture. If they are already nervous or uncomfortable then they will feel even more vulnerable when they need to deal with these 'threats' alone in their home.

Finally, dogs may be bored. Boredom usually affects young or energetic dogs like Cockapoos who still don't know what to do when they are left to play - or relax - alone and they will seek out ways to keep themselves entertained. Like chewing furniture - this is also a calming activity - or exploring the trash. Exercise will help with this.

Dogs will do some of these things some of the time. But when they display this behavior some, or most of the time, then it is likely your dog is suffering from some degree of separation anxiety.

Dogs will get bored when they are left alone. Your dog will sleep – dogs sleep for between to 10 to 14 hours a day - but she will be awake at various points, and she will be looking for something to do.

She might have a sniff around, have a drink or two, and then look for something else to occupy her mind, his energy, and her time.

Dogs like to put things in their mouth, some things fit in their mouths and some things don't. This means that sometimes the mess you discover on returning home is simply a sign of a bored dog and not necessarily one suffering from anxiety.

This doesn't make the experience of returning home any more pleasant, but exercise will help, and finding toys that she can play with will relieve some of that boredom. Other signs, that are more likely to be separation anxiety, are more obvious.

The first thing I noticed was howling when I left the house. I didn't notice it - one of my neighbors told me that when the dog walker dropped them off after their walk they would howl for hours. Until this point, I had no idea.

This not only made me feel like a bad dog parent, but it also made me feel like a bad neighbor.

I would then leave the house for a few minutes and wait outside to see if this was an occasional thing or something they did all the time. Sure enough, after a few minutes, I would hear the howling.

This made it very hard for me to leave the house without worrying about them - and my neighbors. Commonly, the signs of distress manifest almost as soon as you leave the house.

Howling or barking is not the only sign of separation anxiety. Other signs are excessive barking, panting or whining, and indoor accidents. This won't be due to not being housebroken.

Stress can result in either peeing or pooping or both. They may also chew things to calm themselves, scratch at doors or windows and some might try to escape.

They are more likely to be scratching the door that you left from, or the window from where they can see you leave, they might chew something that smells of you - a shoe, sock, or even a magazine.

Signs of general stress in dogs will be panting and pacing and this may well be evident in your dog if she is suffering from separation anxiety.

Is your dog panting when you return home? This might be due to whining and barking while you were gone. You will notice this at other times too.

Separation anxiety is not only when you leave the house and the dog is alone. It can also be when dogs become anxious when they are not seated near you or can't see you even if you arc still at home.

Does your dog follow you around and want to sit beside you all the time? Does she sit against your legs or feet (this way she will know as soon as you move)?

What happens when you leave? Is it only you that your dog is focused on (if you share your home with family). In some cases, it doesn't matter if she is with another person in the home when you leave - it is you that matters to her.

If you share your home and want to find this out, simply have a friend or another family member stay with her (with some treats) and leave the house. How does she react? Does she ignore the treats and look for you and if she does, for how long for? Or does she settle down with the other person and enjoy her treats?

If you are not sure how your dog is reacting when you leave then it is useful to record your dog when you are not there. What does he do when you leave? Does he go to the door for a few minutes - how long? Take note of everything you can see and what he does. This is one of the best ways to find out what is happening when you are gone.

Signs of anxiety

Does your dog start to behave differently as you get ready to leave, either before you have started to get ready or when you are getting ready to leave? My dogs started to react to me picking up my coat or my car keys. If I was going on a trip - which might only be once every few months, one of my dogs would immediately start to pace around and look 'sad' as soon as I got a suitcase out.

The first thing to do is to take notice of their behavior and try and think about if it has changed and why it might have changed. What changes have you made, if any?

Notice how much and how often your dog is following you (even if she is a new puppy). If it's an older dog try to think back to any changes - is she sitting beside you more often, following your more than she used to? Is there any other reason or a point in time that you can identify?

The solution to this part of their behavior is to slowly build them up to being comfortable with you not being beside or near them so that they get used to your absence and learn (or re-learn) that you come back.

It is perfectly natural for dogs to show some anxiety - so don't over-react or worry about it. But if they do suffer from anxiety or nervousness, it is more likely they will also suffer from separation anxiety.

Sometimes any or some of the signs can be there for other reasons so if you are worried at all just check with your veterinarian.

Punishment Won't Work

Before we talk about all the things that can be done to help with separation anxiety, it is useful to understand why punishment just won't work.

Have you ever taken your dog over to the 'scene of the crime' and pointed at it? I have done this and we all will have done this or be tempted to do it.

Notice that the dog appears to look guilty and might cower. We, as humans, project our interpretation to this behavior, and assume that the dog is noticing what it has done and feels 'guilty' about it.

This is not what is happening. What we see as 'looking guilty' is appeasement behavior. It can be a way that your dog is releasing tension to try and get rid of their fear. The cowering, flat ears and tail between the legs, or looking away, is your dog trying to placate you.

The dog will know that she emptied the trash all over the kitchen floor and dragged some of it into other rooms, but it won't connect what she has done wrong minutes or hours later.

All your dog will know is that you are not happy and she will pick this up from you and be fearful, and will try to placate you but she won't know what she has done. She only knows that you are unhappy right now. No matter how much you point at that mess your dog is not going to know why you are angry with her - and that anger will be scary to her.

Dogs won't associate something done hours or even minutes ago with the here-and-now. No matter how much we tell them, they simply won't understand what is going on with us and why we are making them scared.

This all means that punishment when you return home because you have encountered a mess, will make your dog stressed about you coming home. She will already have been stressed about you leaving, and she will have been stressed while you were away. Punishment when you return home can make any anxiety worse.

Just remember, your dog has not done this to deliberately annoy you nor to 'get back' at you. Dogs just don't think like that. They did it because they were stressed and anxious or bored and they tried to use that pent-up energy.

They might look 'guilty' when you return because they have learned that they got into trouble the last time you came back - so they appease you as soon as you return.

But they are doing this because when you return, they sometimes get punished, so they react to prevent it as much as they can.

Preparation

It's a good idea to get your puppy used to being separated from you when they are young. Even if you don't expect to be away from them often, there will be times when you will need to be.

Teaching your puppy not to fear this absence, and to let them know that they can be relaxed when you are not there, is one of the best things you can do for both your puppy, and for yourself.

If your puppy can get used to being left for short periods when she is young, then she is more likely to grow up feeling relaxed and comfortable when she is left on her own for a period of time or part of the day.

Getting her used to not being beside you

These are all really simple things to do and are obvious once you know them. You will need to do this slowly, teaching them bit by bit over time.

The first 3 basic steps that you need to take are the following ones.

1.Pick the room you want your puppy or dog to be in when you are not in the house - either in their basket, bed, or crate. Decide which room this is going to be as early as you can.

2.Once you decide on the location, start getting them used to being in this room - don't wait until the time when you are going to leave the house.

3.Spend time with your puppy in this room - you want them to understand it is not a punishment 'place' or a place that is apart from you, but a part of their household. For example if it is the kitchen and her crate is in the kitchen, have her go into the crate while you are also in the kitchen or create an area that you can block off (and have her crate in).

4. Once you have picked the room that you want your puppy to stay in when you leave the house, create a gate to the room or area by making a barrier so that your puppy can still see you. Again, for example, if the crate is in the kitchen, close the door but remain in the kitchen having a coffee or cooking or just reading. As long as she can see you. Remember not to interact with your puppy when she is there - just go about doing things as normal.

You are aiming to spend time like this and in this room when you are **not** about to leave, spend time there during the day, or when you are training them so that this becomes a place that you are a part of too. You want being in this room and apart from you as a part of their normal day ie. there is no stress for them in not being beside you all the time.

To achieve this you need to start the next stage of their training.

Initially you are going to close the gate but remain beside it. Do this for 2 or 3 minutes but, if your dog starts to get stressed, just calmly let them out.

Keep building their confidence and slowly make the time longer. Start moving around and doing other things as you build up the time and distance. At this point, you will always be in sight.

If they start to get anxious just move forward or return to the point where they were comfortable. Once they are comfortable with the distance, start to move out of sight to another room for a few minutes, and then repeat the process of stretching the time. Begin by moving to the door of the room.

Then move into another room out of sight (but they will still be able to hear and smell you). Return after a few minutes, and then repeat building up the time as you go along.

Finally, go to the main door and go outside for a few minutes. Once again, repeat the process of increasing the time you are away and check how your dog is reacting.

If there are signs of stress or anxiety just go back a couple of steps and begin building up your dog's confidence once again. Keep the time as short as you need to, it can start with as little as 5 or 10 seconds, and build the time based on your dog's response.

From the very start let the dog know that the place you have chosen is their safe place. Keep all their things in this room and place their bed or crate in here as soon as you can, along with some toys.

If you are using a crate, keep the crate door open - let them get used to going in and out of the crate and choosing to do so.

Get some chew toys for them. Chew toys are good because chewing is calming action (and it's why they chew things they shouldn't). You could also put an item of your clothing in the room so that they can more easily smell you and feel more secure.

The chew toys help your dog use their mind to try and work out how to get the food or treat removed. Giving a reason for dogs to exercise their mind keeps them busy and happily occupied. A Kong is a great chew toy to use because, as well as the chewing, the fun of getting the treats or food out of the inside of the Kong exercises their mind.

Put on some sound - like a radio talk station. Not at a high volume - you only want to muffle any unexpected sounds.

This helps my dogs. I use either the television news or a talk radio channel because these shows are unlikely to have sudden noises. Whatever you choose, make it something that you listen to so that they are familiar with it.

Your dog will be paying attention to any noise they hear, so this can help disguise some of the day-to-day noises that might go on outside (or inside) your home. It is useful to do this as soon as you begin the training to get them used to it. .

Try to teach your dog not to follow you all the time in the home. You want her to feel comfortable being in another room from you. Don't force this or make her feel stressed about it. You can do this by playing a game with her but you won't be able to do this until you have taught her the 'stay' cue.

Ask her to remain in one room while you move to another, then come back. If she stays where she was, come back and give her a reward. Remember, when you come back not to increase or cause excitement, you want to keep her calm. This can be a great game for your dog and she will enjoy it as much as you enjoy the results of it.

When you are ready to start the next phase of actually leaving the house there are a few more things you can do to keep your dog calm while you are out.

Leaving and returning

Start by leaving the house for a minute, 2 minutes, 3 minutes, and so on, and try and return before they are anxious. If you can, then leave for longer and build up to an hour and so on. If you notice they are not comfortable, then go back to the point when they were, and start from there again. Build the time up again.

Aim to build the routine - perhaps a treat as you leave. But don't kiss and cuddle them and make a fuss with gestures and by your comments. Try and make it as normal and calm as possible.

Of everything I did to help with Barney's separation anxiety, this was the single and most effective technique. It seems so simple yet it seemed to (and still does) calm her. I stopped saying goodbye or paying attention when I left. I just put on my coat, made no fuss at all, and left calmly.

Once you start leaving altogether, do so for short periods at the start if you can, and build up the time to 2, 3 and 4 hours. Do everything as normal and as they are now used to - and make sure they have something to play with or to eat.

Ideally, don't leave your dog alone for more than 4 hours. If you can ask a neighbor or a friend to visit - one your dog might know - or a dog walker. If you are able, come home from work for lunch.

You might start to notice that your dog starts to get anxious when you put on your shoes or coat or if you pick up keys or a bag.

If they start to react to these signs then start training them to get used to these things. Put on your shoes or coat or grab your keys but don't leave. Do something else or sit down and relax (or watch the TV). Keep doing this during the day so that they don't associate these things with your departure.

For example, one of my dogs would start jumping around as soon as I got my boots out. Initially, I put them on in another room, and then I realized I had to be in control of their reaction. I put the boots on then didn't leave (you can do this with keys/coats etc, pick them up or put it on and just sit for a while).

You can also try body-blocking. I used this with the younger dog, Barney (he was more excitable). As soon as he started to get agitated as the boots or coat came out I interrupted his behavior by standing up straight and then asking him to go to his basket. It's important not to be angry - they aren't doing anything wrong - you just want them to do something else so let them know what that is e.g. go to their crate or their basket.

You might need to go back a few paces in the separation training from time-to-time, as you are building their confidence and their sense of 'normal'. Just go back to the point where your dog was last comfortable.

Take this slowly - leave and come back. Build their knowledge and confidence. Having them exercised will help reduce their energy levels so remember to make sure they have had a walk and have been fed. This will make her tired.

You can also try giving them a favorite treat. This might help them associate your departure with something they can look forward to. Someone I know uses a hollowed-out bone with frozen dog food inside (they put the dog food in the bone then freeze it). You could do the same with a Kong.

When you return, don't get them excited with happy cries of "hello!". Don't over-excite them, or over-reward them when you come back. Just arrive home and then ignore them for 5 minutes. You need to make the exit and return a very normal thing rather than any kind of event to be excited about.

If they have done something wrong on your return don't punish them or shout at them. They won't understand why.

Summary

- Don't make a fuss of your dog when you leave. Don't kiss them and say 'goodbye'.
- Leave calmly.
- Give them their favorite treat as you leave - give them something to chew on.
- Make sure they have been exercised.
- Don't excite them as soon as you return home, wait a few minutes before greeting them.(These steps were the most effective things that I did to help my dog with separation).

Leaving when using a crate

When you put your dog in their crate (if you use a crate) before you leave then don't close the door right away. Put them in and wait until they calm down or lie down.

This might take a few minutes or more so do something else and give them time to relax and be calm. Close and open the door a few times if you like, but wait until they lie down before you close the door.

Don't bribe them into the crate with a treat and then immediately shut the door - just take your time, and let them take their time to get

Once they are comfortable in their space and their room then you can start moving away using the methods detailed in the first step.

Some other useful tips

1. Exercise is an important part of curing separation anxiety.

A 2015 study by PLoS One found that dogs with noise sensitivity and separation anxiety had less daily exercise. This suggests that exercise is one of the biggest things you can do to prevent or improve separation anxiety in your dog. You need to make sure your pet gets lots of exercise every day because a tired, happy dog will be less stressed when you leave.

The study also found that dogs that were exercised off-leash were less likely to suffer from separation anxiety or fear around noise. The likely reason for this is that being on a leash, partly on a leash, or running free, has an impact on the amount of exercise a dog has.

2. A dog whines when it starts to get tense or excited - think of as them releasing their energy. Sometimes they whine because they want something - if this is the case, they will make it obvious what they want. If you notice this and the reason is not obvious then try and work out why it might be excited and calm them down before the excitement level rises.

3. If you have multiple household members - try and share the dog equally amongst everyone - so the dog doesn't focus all their attention onto one person. If there are more members then one

can leave and he dog will worry less. Research shows that dogs in multiple person households are more likely to suffer from separation anxiety – I had expected it to be the other way around.

10 Steps to help Separation Anxiety

1. Create a physical barrier between the room you want them to remain in and the room you are in - make this something they can see you through.
2. Put their bedding or basket in this room along with any of their toys and the bowls.
3. Put on some sound - like a radio talk station. Not at a high volume - you only want to muffle any unexpected sounds.
4. Teach your dog not to follow you all the time in the home.
5. Don't make a fuss of your dog when you leave. Don't cuddle and kiss them and say 'goodbye'
6. Leave calmly
7. Give them their favorite treat as you leave - give them something to chew on
8. Make sure they have been exercised
9. When you return don't over-excite your dog as soon as you arrive home (if there is a mess, don't punish your dog)
10. Wait a few minutes before you acknowledge them and say hello.

Chapter 14
How to find a breeder

Reputable - or ethical - breeders invest in good quality dog food, they have good veterinary care, they tend to only breed their females up to twice year and they work to established breeding plans. All of this means that they spend more on the care of the dogs which is why the cost will be higher. If you find a breeder and they offer you a low price then you can be pretty sure they are not reputable.

You should expect to be asked questions about the puppy's care and you may be asked to sign a contract that deals with health and should include a return to breeder clause that means you will return the puppy if you can no longer care for him or her.

If you are not quizzed about how you will care for your Cockapoo puppy then it is likely, no matter how high the cost, that you are not dealing with a reputable breeder.

Other things that can help identify a reputable breeder will be if they have extensive knowledge of Cockapoos and their generations, they will ideally work with a vet, undertake health screening, and if you have been on a wait list this is another good sign.

They should also be able to show genetic screening and the lineage of your puppy (which should be extensive).

How to recognise a puppy farm

When you are buying a puppy, you might not recognise that you're buying from a puppy farm. Many of these types of sellers are experienced and go to extremes to cover up what they really are.

A puppy farm isn't always obvious, so look out for some important signs at each stage of purchasing your puppy.

Advertising

If you see an advert online, check how many other ads the seller is running. A puppy farm is more than likely to be advertising more than one litter and may also be advertising different breeds. To check, you can google the number in the advert to find out how often it is being used and for what.

If the advert claims the puppy has been vaccinated and the puppy is under 6 weeks old then this would indicate the advert is from a puppy farm. (Always request written evidence that your puppy and his mother have been vaccinated).

If your puppy comes with a passport (and has been imported), make sure that your puppy is 12 weeks old. They should be this age to qualify for a passport. If there is no passport then it is more likely your puppy has come from a country with poor legislation around puppy farming.

Always make sure that you see the puppy at her home and where she has been born.

Make sure the seller does not have other breeds - most breeders specialize in just one breed and should have a depth of knowledge about Cockapoos. A puppy farmer will not have the knowledge so be prepared to ask some questions

Make sure that you see the mum and note how the mother reacts to the seller as well as the overall condition of the mum. She should not be wary of the breeder. But also note how she reacts to the puppy. You want to be sure that she is the mother and not another dog that is being presented to you as the mum.

As noted above, the breeder should be asking you lots of questions to make sure you can look after your new puppy. If they are not interested in you and how you will care for the puppy, then they are unlikely to be interested in the puppy's welfare.

Puppy farms often prefer to deal with cash and do not offer refunds or have a no returns policy. You should always seek a puppy contract that lays out the responsibilities and a returns policy.

Health Clearances

A good breeder will show you health clearances for both of your puppy's parents. Health clearances prove that a dog has been tested for, and cleared for, a particular condition.

Liver disease has been mentioned previously and it is a condition that is becoming more prevalent in Cocker Spaniels: chronic active hepatitis and copper toxicosis (poisoning. Both conditions may or may not be genetic and, at this point, no one is certain. More research is needed, but meanwhile ask your Cockapoo breeder about the parent Cocker's liver history.

Health clearances are not issued to dogs younger than 2 years of age. That's because some health problems don't appear until a dog reaches full maturity. For this reason, it's often recommended that dogs not be bred until they are two or three years old.

Test and examples of organisation who certificate

- Progressive Retinal Atrophy (RDA) - Canine Eye Registry Foundation (both parents)
- Glaucoma (both parents)
- Hip/Elbow Dysplasia (Cocker Spaniel) - Orthopaedic Foundation for Animals (OFA)/BVA/Kennel Club
- Familial nephropathy (kidney problems) – Cocker Spaniel
- Von Willebrand Disease (Poodle) - Auburn University

Chapter 15
Conclusion and Summary

There is probably no better word to describe a Cockapoo other than 'cheeky'. Their little round adorable faces will be impossible to get annoyed with and they will forever be looking into your eyes with a lovable, determined, self-assured smile. How they love you!

But, as my grandmother would say 'you would let her get away with murder', and you will, and you will still give her a kiss and a hug after giving her into trouble for being 'naughty'.

And naughty they are. But that is the fun of them and it's up to you to train them so that you can all can laugh and love their naughtiness, and ensure that it is never a risk to them.

The Cockapoo is intelligent, she will be easy to train with positive reinforcement. She is a great family and companion dog. She is friendly, she is loving and you will be the centre of her world. She will generally like other dogs and children (preferably older children) but might be prone to separation anxiety but all of these things can be dealt with with a little bit of patient training.

Don't worry if it takes longer than you imagined. It's not a competition and every dog and every family is different. There is no hard and fast rule of how long some things can take. Try to enjoy it, and take lots of pictures and video's - they grow up so fast!

Chapter 16
Need more help?

I just came across this fantastic (and free) online workshop on training your dog to become as well-behaved as a service dog.

I loved the workshop so much that I wanted to share it with you immediately.

Check out the free workshop here

The workshop is designed to help "normal" dogs like yours have the same level of calmness, obedience and impulse control as service dogs.

It's being conducted by Dr. Alexa Diaz (one of the top service dog trainers in the U.S.) and Eric Presnall (host of the hit Animal Planet TV show "Who Let the Dogs Out").

Frankly, the techniques described in the workshop are fairly groundbreaking - I haven't seen anyone else talk of these techniques.

This is because it's the first time ever (at least that I know of) that anyone has revealed the techniques used by the service dog training industry to train service dogs.

And more importantly, how any "regular" dog owner can apply the same techniques to train their own dogs to become as well-trained as service dogs.

It's not a live workshop - rather, it's a pre-recorded workshop, which means that you can watch it at your convenience.

However, while the workshop is free, I am not sure whether it's going to be online for too long, so please check it out as soon as you can.

Here's the link again.

Or you can use this QR code.

Leave A Review

As an independent publisher with a small marketing budget, reviews are my livelihood on this platform. If you enjoyed this book, I'd really appreciate it if you leave your honest feedback. If you think this book can help other Cockapoo owners then please let them know by leaving a review. You can do this by clicking the link to leave a review. I love hearing from my readers, and I personally read every single review. The address for UK and US review links are below:

UK: https://www.amazon.co.uk/review/create-review/?asin=1739983955

US: http://amazon.com/review/create-review/asin=1739983955

If you want to talk to other Cockapoo owners and ask or share advice then you can join the private Facebook Group here:

https://www.facebook.com/groups/cockapoocommunity

Leave A Review

More Books From Twenty Dogs

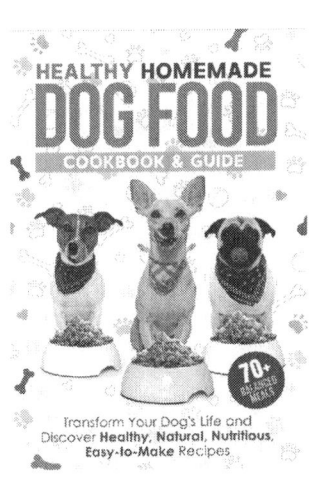

www.amazon.com/dp/B0C52MWPLM

www.amazon.co.uk/dp/B0C52MWPLM

Healthy Homemade Dog Food Amazon Link (US)

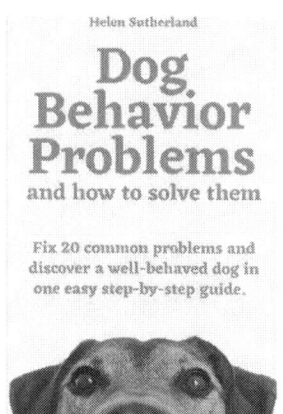

www.amazon.com/dp/B0C526728C

www.amazon.co.uk/dp/B0C526728C

Dog Behavior Problems and How To Solve Them (US)

Resources and Citations

Alt, K. (2020, August 14). *Am I Ready For A Dog? How To Be A Responsible Dog Owner.* Canine Journal. https://www.ca-ninejournal.com/am-i-ready-for-a-dog

Animal Poison Control. (n.d.). The American Society for the Prevention of Cruelty to Animals® (ASPCA®). https://www.aspca.org/pet-care/animal-poison-control/people-foods-avoid-feeding-your-pets

Answer These 5 Questions to Find the Right Dog For You. (2017, November 2). American Kennel Club. https://www.akc.org/expert-advice/lifestyle/answer-5-questions-find-right-dog/

Blue Cross For Pets. (n.d.). Blue Cross For Pets. https://www.bluecross.org.uk/advice/dog

Committee on Nutrient Requirements of Dogs and Cats. (2006). *Your Dog's Nutritional Needs. Retrieved.* (2006). Https://Www.Nap.Edu. https://www.nap.edu/resource/10668/dog_nutrition_final_fix.pdf

Resources and Citations

What Size Dog Crate Do You Need? (n.d.). Cooper's Crates (www.Cooperscrates.Com). https://cooperscrates.com/pages/selecting-the-correct-kennel-size

Your Complete Guide to First-Year Puppy Vaccinations. (2021, February 5). American Kennel Club (Www.Akc.Org). https://www.akc.org/expert-advice/health/puppy-shots-complete-guide

Gibeault, MSc, CPDT, S. (2021, February 3). *How To Teach Your Dog To Sit.* Https://Www.Akc.Org/. https://www.akc.org/expert-advice/training/how-to-teach-your-dog-to-sit/

Madson, MA, CBCC-KA, CPDT-KA, C. (2020, July 25). *How To Teach Your Dog To Come When Called.* Https://Www.Preventivevet.Com/. https://www.preventivevet.com/dogs/how-to-teach-your-dog-to-come-when-called

Recall Training. (n.d.). Https://Www.Doglistener.Co.Uk. https://www.doglistener.co.uk/behavioural/recall_training.shtml

Simply Behaviour. (n.d.). *Simply Behaviour.* Http://Www.Simplybehaviour.Com/. http://www.simplybehaviour.com/

Yin, D. S. (n.d.). *Teaching Rover To Race To You In Cue.* Cattledog Publishing. https://drsophiayin.com/blog/entry/teaching_rover_to_race_to_you_on_cue/

https://www.thelabradorsite.com/teaching-a-dog-to-heel/

Salonen, M., Sulkama, S., Mikkola, S. *et al. Prevalence, comorbidity, and breed differences in canine anxiety in 13,700 Finnish pet dogs. Sci Rep* **10,** 2962 (2020). https://doi.org/10.1038/s41598-020-59837-z

Barbara L. Sherman, Daniel S. Mills, *Canine Anxieties and Phobias: An Update on Separation Anxiety and Noise Aversions, Veterinary Clinics of North America*: Small Animal Practice, Volume 38, Issue 5, 2008, Pages 1081-1106, ISSN 0195-5616, https://doi.org/10.1016/j.cvsm.2008.04.012

Blue Cross For Pets, Retrieved from https://www.bluecross.org.uk/pet-advice/home-alone-separation-anxiety-dogs

Tiira, Katriina & Lohi, Hannes. (2015). *Early Life Experiences and Exercise Associate with Canine Anxieties. PloS one.* 10. e0141907. 10.1371/journal.pone.0141907. Retrieved from https://www.researchgate.net/publication/283492761_Early_Life_Experiences_and_Exercise_Associate_with_Canine_Anxieties

Dog Psychology 101, https://dogpsychology101.com/

Pet Poison helpline https://www.petpoisonhelpline.com/pet-owners/emergency/

Debra C. Sellon, Katherine Martucci, John R. Wenz, Denis J. Marcellin-Little, Michelle Powers, Kimberley L. Cullen. A survey of risk factors for digit injuries among dogs training and competing in agility events. J Am Vet Med Assoc 2018;252:75-83

The Kennel Club. (n.d.). *Why does my dog eat poop.* Https://Www.Thekennelclub.Org.Uk. https://www.thekennelclub.org.uk/health-and-dog-care/health/health-and-care/a-z-of-health-and-care-issues/why-does-my-dog-eat-poop/

dogtime.com/dog-breeds/cockapoo. (n.d.). Dogtime.Com. https://dogtime.com/dog-breeds/cockapoo#/slide/1

British Cockapoo Society. (n.d.). British Cockapoo Society. https://www.britishcockapoosociety.com

Debra C. Sellon, Katherine Martucci, John R. Wenz, Denis J. Marcellin-Little, Michelle Powers, Kimberley L. Cullen. (2018). A survey of risk factors for digit injuries among dogs training and competing in agility events. *PubMed: J Am Vet Med Association*. https://doi.org/10.2460/javma.252.1.75

Dew claws. (n.d.). Mill Creek Family Farms. https://www.mill creekfamilyfarms.com/dew-claws

Jennifer L. Manning-Paro. (2020, December). *Canine Front Limb Dewclaw Removal and the Resulting Carpal Injury and Arthritis Risks*. Hands of Grace Animal Massage and Body-work. https://www.handsofgraceanimalmassageandbodywork. com/blog/canine-front-limb-dewclaw-removal-and-the-result ing-carpal-injury-and-arthritis-risks

M J Schmidt 1, A C Neumann, K H Amort, K Failing, M Kramer. (2011). Cephalometric measurements and determination of general skull type of Cavalier King Charles Spaniels. *National Library of Medicine*. https://doi.org/10.1111/j.1740-8261.2011.01825.x

The Natural Dog - A Guide to Raw Diet adn Health the Natural Way. (n.d.). Rawfed Dogs - The Natural Dog. http:// rawfeddogs.org/rawguide

Made in United States
Troutdale, OR
04/17/2024

19239050R10099